WITHDRAWN

D1570293

Forget Dieting!

Forget Dieting!

It's All about Data-Driven Fueling

Candice P. Rosen

ROWMAN & LITTLEFIELD
Lanham • Boulder • New York • London

Published by Rowman & Littlefield
An imprint of The Rowman & Littlefield Publishing Group, Inc.
4501 Forbes Boulevard, Suite 200, Lanham, Maryland 20706
www.rowman.com

6 Tinworth Street, London SE11 5AL, United Kingdom

British Library Cataloguing in Publication Information Available

Library of Congress Cataloging-in-Publication Data
Names: Rosen, Candice P., 1954– author.
Title: Forget dieting! : it's all about data-driven fueling / Candice P.
  Rosen.
Description: Lanham : Rowman & Littlefield, [2020] | Includes
  bibliographical references and index. | Summary: "The dieting industry
  has done little to decrease obesity and its associated health issues.
  Candice Rosen encourages us to Forget Dieting! and tune into our
  bodies to discover the foods that work best for us. By focusing on blood
  sugar, readers will learn to listen to their bodies to achieve lasting
  weight loss, increased energy, and better sleep"— Provided by
  publisher.
Identifiers: LCCN 2019041732 (print) | LCCN 2019041733 (ebook) |
  ISBN 9781538131497 (cloth) | ISBN 9781538136317 (epub)
Subjects: LCSH: Reducing diets—Health aspects. | Nutrition.
Classification: LCC RM222.2 .R64748 2020 (print) | LCC RM222.2
  (ebook) | DDC 613.2/5—dc23
LC record available at https://lccn.loc.gov/2019041732
LC ebook record available at https://lccn.loc.gov/2019041733

This book is dedicated to my reasons for being,
Melissa, Jennifer, Natalie, and Nicholas,
and my wish upon a star, Lillian Marlene Mack

To my mother and father, who provided a solid
foundation and encouraged critical thinking—
to always question and never take anything at face value

To my husband Steve for supporting my evolution

And to my clients, who place their faith in me

Health Disclaimer

This publication is intended to provide helpful tips, advice, and suggestions to assist readers with interest in obtaining information regarding dietary and activity changes. It is not intended to diagnose, treat, cure, or prevent any health condition or concern.

The information provided in this book should not be interpreted as a substitute for physician consultation, evaluation, or treatment. Nothing written in this book should be construed as medical advice or diagnosis. Before beginning any diet and/or exercise program, always consult with your physician or primary health-care provider to ensure your health and safety. Any suggestions or inferences drawn from this book should be reviewed with a licensed medical professional before implementation. The author and publisher will not be held responsible for individuals who carry out intended or unintended harm to themselves or other individuals.

The author, publisher, its agents, and its representatives shall not be held responsible for any information interpreted as such by any readers. The author, publisher, its agents, and its representatives specifically disclaim all responsibility for any liability, loss of risk, personal or otherwise, which may be incurred as a consequence, directly or indirectly, from the use or application of any contents of this book. The statements made in this book have not been evaluated by the Food and Drug Administration of the United States of America.

Contents

PREFACE — xi

NOTE TO THE READER: CHALLENGING A
DELUDED NATION — xvii

ACKNOWLEDGMENTS — xxi

Section I: The Basics — 1

CHAPTER 1   What Happens When I Eat? — 3

CHAPTER 2   How Do High Glucose and Insulin
Affect Weight and Health? — 8

CHAPTER 3   Hormones, Stress, and Weight — 15

Section II: Data-Driven Fueling — 27

CHAPTER 4   Data-Driven Fueling Guidelines — 29

CHAPTER 5   The Data-Driven Fueling Lifestyle — 33

CHAPTER 6   The Data-Driven Fueling Program — 44

CHAPTER 7   A Day in the Life of Data-Driven Fueling — 48

CHAPTER 8   Data-Driven Fueling Calendar — 52

Section III: Other Issues Affecting Health   57

CHAPTER 9   Behavior Modification   59

CHAPTER 10   Movement   72

CHAPTER 11   The Importance of Sleep   78

CHAPTER 12   Sabotage   88

CHAPTER 13   Addictions Other Than Food:
             Drugs and Alcohol   96

Section IV: Data-Driven Fueling Toolbox   101

CHAPTER 14   Basic Food Combining   103

CHAPTER 15   The Anatomy of a Meal   111

CHAPTER 16   Meal Choices   119

CHAPTER 17   The Importance of Journaling
             and Meal Discovery Cards   125

CHAPTER 18   What to Do with a High Glucose Number   133

CHAPTER 19   Vitamins   136

CHAPTER 20   What to Do If You Hit a Plateau   141

CHAPTER 21   Eating Out of Your Element:
             College and Travel   144

CHAPTER 22   Recipes for Meals and Liquid Fasts   149

FINAL THOUGHTS   167

NOTES   169

BIBLIOGRAPHY   175

INDEX   179

ABOUT THE AUTHOR   191

Preface

Forget Dieting! Who wants or likes to diet? I don't! There are thousands of diets worldwide. I read somewhere that on any given day, one in three women and one in four men are dieting. What does that tell you? Essentially, that diets don't work!

Diets equal restraint, self-denial, major workouts, abstinence, restrictions, and anticipated loss of enjoyment.

Well, no more. I don't diet, and I don't work out vigorously. Instead, I follow a Data-Driven Fueling lifestyle based on solid empirical information from my body. It's really about personalized precision nutrition: I know exactly what foods/fuels work best for my body, and I want to help you learn too!

I am a registered nurse, social worker, certified health counselor, and the author of *The Pancreatic Oath* (a diet book that details how blood glucose affects weight and health). *Forget Dieting!*—my third book—is different. I often talk too much. I often explain too much. A dear friend said to me, "Keep it simple, please!" So, I have really tried to do that with this book.

Forget Dieting! will convince you that you have the power to achieve sustainable, long-term weight loss and transform your health. I know you've heard it before, but trust me—you really do. But first you have to understand how food affects your weight and your health. Once you understand that, you'll be able to say, "F dieting!"

It took me a long time to understand and accept this fact. For years, I thought my size was embedded in my DNA. I was born into an ethnic family that equated appetite with health. The more you ate, the healthier you were. Skimping on food was unheard of.

My whole family has a history of weight issues, heart disease, and diabetes—commonly referred to as "medical baggage." I was convinced that this baggage would be my burden to carry and pass on. I now know that isn't true. In fact, I don't have heart disease or diabetes and weigh less now than I did in high school!

I believe the reasons for my family's health issues were misinformation and a general lack of understanding about how the body (especially the pancreas) functions. My mom self-soothed with food. She was incorrectly informed that Stella Doro dietetic cookies, along with Tab and Diet Pepsi, were healthy choices for a type 2 diabetic. She believed that the drug Metformin allowed her to eat whatever she wanted. Her view of "healthy" was skewed, and consequently so was mine.

Although I was never obese, as a nonpregnant adult, I was about thirty-five pounds overweight. I hid it well by wearing oversized clothes and lots of black. I fooled myself into thinking that there was nothing I could do. I believed that my size was the by-product of being the mother of four children, or that I had a genetic issue, and I was convinced that I was eating healthily. I was taught that meals should include a protein, a starch, salad, lots of bread, and a homemade dessert. My mom believed this was not only a healthy meal but also a loving meal.

Before I started Data-Driven Fueling, I tried what seemed like every diet out there: Weight Watchers, liquid protein, cabbage soup, the Zone, Atkins, SlimFast, Scarsdale, the grapefruit diet, and even diet pills. Each attempt to lose weight was prompted by a special event: a reunion, a wedding, or a vacation. I would lose twenty pounds through restricted calories and draining workouts, only to gain back what I had lost—and then some. Regaining what you have lost is frustrating and depressing. According to a University of California, Los Angeles review of more than thirty studies, 83 percent of dieters who achieved their goals gained back all their weight and more.[1]

The weight-loss market is a $66 billion industry, with dropping pounds being the ultimate goal. Yet more than 70 percent of U.S. adults remain either overweight or obese.[2] It doesn't make sense. I hated dieting, and I hated complicated diet programs. To me, counting calories, points, carbohydrates, or fats, along with keeping track of workouts or steps, was time consuming and overwhelming.

With that in mind, I developed a program that I know works. Called Data-Driven Fueling, it is a sister plan to my Pancreatic Nutritional Program. This program is about a simple and long-lasting lifestyle change that is rooted in data.

Your body is hardwired to heal itself and maintain an appropriate weight. Your mind, body, and spirit are intertwined. I believe in the practice of *self-health*. In this practice, you are your primary caregiver; your physician is your secondary caregiver.

My hypothesis is that many noncommunicable diseases (NCDs), such as high blood pressure, high cholesterol, obesity, type 2 diabetes, polycystic ovarian syndrome, metabolic syndrome, insulin resistance, low testosterone, renal issues, and even some cancers, stem from pancreatic abuse. *What is pancreatic abuse? Any time you raise your blood sugar over 100 milligrams per deciliter (mg/dL) ninety minutes after you eat a meal or a snack, you should expect weight gain and NCDs. The goal is to keep your blood sugar between 70 and 100 mg/dL.*

I'm going to show you a very simple way to lose weight and heal yourself. This book is not going to be filled with excessive studies; you are going to have to trust what I tell you. Please don't rush through *Forget Dieting!* It's loaded with important information that will enable you to weave the Forget Dieting! lifestyle into your being. It's a process. My personal experience; the experiences of my clients, family, and friends; and the success of a recent study of the Pancreatic Nutrition Program at City of Hope Comprehensive Cancer Center (Duarte, California) all confirm that protecting your pancreas by maintaining normal glucose levels works.

Study Results

Pancreatic Nutrition Program (PNP): A Novel Weight-Reduction Program for Breast Cancer Survivors

BACKGROUND: Breast cancer survivors have a high prevalence of metabolic dysfunction—characterized by high glucose and weight gain. Regardless of menopausal status, overweight and obese women are at increased risk for developing breast cancer and those who are diagnosed with breast cancer experience adverse cancer-related outcomes. The underlying principle of the Pancreatic Nutrition Program (PNP) is that bio-individualized healthy food choices—eating the correct foods and food combinations for an individual's body—can minimize fluctuations in insulin by keeping blood glucose regulated (70–100 mg/dL) and this will promote sustained weight loss, improved health, and quality of life.

METHODS: The primary endpoint was change in body weight at 24 weeks post-PNP. The study was powered to detect a 10% loss of weight from baseline. Secondary endpoints included change in: glucose levels, insulin resistance, body composition, body chemistry, physical fitness, biological markers, quality of life, and compliance. Postmenopausal, nondiabetic breast cancer survivors (stages I–III) within 5 years of completion of treatment who had a body mass index of 25–33 kg/m2 were recruited. For the first 12 weeks, patients wore a glucometer (Abbott), which recorded glucose every 15 minutes continuously, and kept a food journal. During weekly meetings, glucometer data was reviewed with journal entries to identify food choices and combinations that would keep the subject's glucose levels between 70–100 mg/dL. At the end of the 12-weeks, the weekly meetings and glucometer were discontinued and patients were expected to maintain the PNP for an additional 12 weeks. Study endpoints were measured at baseline, 12-week and 24-week visits.

RESULTS: Of the 21 patients enrolled in the study, 12 were non-Hispanic Caucasian, 5 were Hispanic, 2 were African-American, and 2 were Asian. The median age was 56 years (43–76 years). Twenty were estrogen-receptor positive, 18 progesterone-receptor positive, and 8 were HER2/neu positive. The mean body weight at baseline was 170.9 lbs

(±20.4 lbs). Two patients dropped out prior to 12-weeks and 1 developed recurrent disease. Among the 18 eligible women who completed the first 12 weeks, the median weight loss at 12-weeks was 10.1 lbs (1.5–19.6 lbs). The median waist circumference lost was 2.5 inches (gain of 0.4 inches–loss of 5.5 inches). Among the women whose total cholesterol was above 200 mg/dL, 71 percent reduced their cholesterol below 200 mg/dL by 12-weeks. All women who had triglyceride levels above 150 mg/dL reduced their levels below 150 mg/dL by 12-weeks. Likewise, among women who were identified as being pre-diabetic based on fasting glucose or hemoglobin A1c levels, all were within normal range at 12-weeks. 6-month testing will be completed in August. Among the 15 women eligible for 6-month testing, 8 (53%) completed the testing. Of those, 7 (88%) maintained their positive results.

CONCLUSIONS: Bio-individualized food choices based on glucose response combined with culturally-sensitive nutrition counseling may provide a feasible mechanism for sustainable weight loss in a population at high-risk of metabolic dysfunction. However, to increase adherence, a tapering strategy should be developed after the first 12-weeks of health counseling.

Your body is a living miracle. As an organic machine, it requires daily maintenance and proper fuel to function at its optimum level. I believe the body has the ability to heal itself if given the proper tools: wholesome, nutritious, responsibly grown, pancreas-friendly foods and activity.

Let's Forget Dieting! and begin Data-Driven Fueling for health and wellness!

Note to the Reader: Challenging a Deluded Nation

In 2016, the Centers for Disease Control stated that 70 percent of Americans are obese or overweight, but only 36 percent think they have a weight problem.[1] Think about it. Close to half the people who are overweight or obese do not believe they are overweight or obese.

America is suffering from body dysmorphia. Many overweight and obese individuals don't look in the mirror and see a serious health issue. They see what they believe to be "normal." They have become desensitized due to the widespread nature of America's weight problem.

The American Society of Clinical Oncology stated in 2016 that obesity has bypassed tobacco as the number one preventable cause of cancers. Cancers fueled by obesity are on the rise among young adults in the United States and are appearing at increasingly younger ages, according to a 2019 analysis released by the American Cancer Society.[2]

If you are overweight or obese, you are at major risk for the following health issues: high blood pressure, type 2 diabetes, stroke, coronary heart disease, gallbladder disease, sleep apnea, osteoarthritis, and generalized body pain. Obesity can also contribute to an overall low quality of life and worsen or increase susceptibility to the development of anxiety and depression.

Like many, I'm deeply saddened about the current obesity and diabetes epidemics in the United States. With so many magazine articles, weight-loss and fitness experts, health tips, and apps to educate and assist in weight loss, why are Americans (especially our children) getting fatter and sicker? Six- to eight-year-olds with obesity are approximately ten times more likely to become obese adults than those with a lower body mass index. A third of the children born in 2000 in this country will develop diabetes during their lifetimes. More than one in four seventeen- to twenty-four-year-olds in the United States are now too heavy to serve in the military, a development that retired military leaders say endangers national security. Since 1980, the obesity prevalence among children and adolescents has almost tripled. Children with obesity are already demonstrating cardiovascular risk factors typically not seen until adulthood. Children with obesity have three times more health-care expenditures than children at healthy weights, costing an estimated $14 billion every year.[3] It is beyond pathetic and tragic. You need to **Forget Dieting!** and think about fueling for weight loss and improved health—if not for yourself, then certainly for your loved ones.

Currently, we are indoctrinated in the idea that body positivity and self-love rest on accepting excess weight. But what does excess weight represent? Typically, excess weight represents present or future poor health. You may be the most handsome guy or the most beautiful gal, but if you are obese, you are putting your body and your health in danger. So no more excuses like "It's because of menopause," "I'm big boned," "My family is overweight," "It's in my genes," "I was born this way," or "It's a thyroid condition." No more pretending. You need to challenge the so-called new normal and get real about your weight and your health! Weight gain and weight loss are elementary. They really are.

What leads to weight gain? Simply put, it's food. Weight gain results from taking in the wrong foods and/or the wrong amount of food for your body, coupled with living a sedentary lifestyle. Your body responds with "I can only use about 10 percent of what you just ate, and because you don't move much, I'll just store the rest of the 90 percent in your face, neck, arms, stomach, butt, and thighs!"

What leads to weight loss? Simply put, weight loss results from taking in the correct foods in appropriate amounts for your body, coupled with movement. Your body responds with "I can use everything you just ate, and because you are moving and not sitting on the couch, I'm forced to go into the storage tanks (face, neck, arms, stomach, butt, and thighs) for the extra fuel." It is the way to lose weight, fuel, and care for your organic machine.

The first step to weight loss and improved health is changing your mind-set about how you approach fueling your body. Don't delude yourself anymore into believing that you have no control over your weight or your health. You do, and I want to help you.

Acknowledgments

I am fortunate to share my beliefs with you about the pancreas and your ability to Forget Dieting! and adapt to a lifestyle of Data-Driven Fueling because of many people. I want to thank my children, who are my greatest joys and biggest supporters: Jennifer, who was my first partner on the path to self-health; Melissa, who exposed me to thought leaders and new ideas about health and wellness; Natalie, who helped with my manuscript and was my willing guinea pig; and Nicholas, who provided valuable exercise information along with insight on stress and motivation. Their opinions, humor, and love are valued beyond measure. I'd also like to thank my husband Steve, a source of support who never complained about the dietary changes in our home.

I am deeply grateful to Nancy Rosenfeld, my literary agent, who believed in me and my message, and my editor, Suzanne Staszak-Silva at Rowman & Littlefield, who took a chance on me. Both women were instrumental in bringing *Forget Dieting!* to publication. I'd also like to thank Patricia Stevenson, senior production editor at Rowman & Littlefield, along with Jennifer Kelland and Charlotte Gosnell. They were patient with this IT-compromised author.

To Sarah Wilkinson and Ariel Guterman, although brief, your assistance is very much appreciated. I am indebted to Dr. Joanne Mortimer for encouraging me to apply for the Circle 1500 grant, which, along with funding from Abbott Labs (thank you Diabetes Division), made my research dream a reality. To Dr. Jessica Clague DeHart, thank you for being my Mini-Me and validating what I witnessed with my clients. The result: the Pancreatic Nutritional Program, a novel weight-reduction program for breast cancer survivors, which was presented at the International Breast Cancer Symposium in San Antonio, Texas, December 2017.

Thank you to Michele Prince for her thoughtful comments and title brainstorming. Thank you also to Lydia Glass for her insight and support.

I am deeply grateful to Joshua Stroud for his technical support and help with formatting.

Throughout my career, I have had the honor and privilege of watching many amazing individuals—clients who have triumphed over illness and weight issues and health-care professionals who were willing to step outside the traditional medical model and explore other treatment options (i.e., the Pancreatic Nutritional Program/Data-Driven Fueling). Every time I work with a client and witness the body's ability to transform when given proper fuel, I am humbled. The human body is like no machine ever created.

My quest is to educate everyone about the pancreas and the role it plays in health and weight. I want to put health back into health care. *Food truly is medicine.*

Section I

The Basics

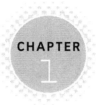

What Happens
When I Eat?

How does your body process the food you eat, and why does it have an effect on your weight and your health? Please read this carefully. Knowing how your organic machine operates every time you eat is critical to Forget Dieting!

Whether you cook at home, eat in a restaurant, order in, or grab food at a drive-thru joint, I'm guessing that you never think about the physiological changes that occur when you eat. I don't know whether individuals think about digestion and absorption of the donut they just ate or how that donut is converted into fuel for their body, their organic living machine. But they should. Most thought processes focus on the intake of food, how it looks and what it tastes like, and some might think about elimination, but I don't believe the majority of people give a hoot about what goes on as it passes from their mouth to their backside.

I'd like to take this opportunity to give you a crash course in digestion. The digestive tract is composed of the mouth, esophagus (muscular tube connecting the throat to the stomach), stomach, small intestine, large intestine, and rectum. The mouth connects with the stomach by way of the pharynx (the throat leading from the mouth and nasal cavity) and esophagus.[1]

Dr. William Beaumont (1785–1853), an army surgeon and the first to observe digestion directly, is considered the father of gastric physiology. Alexis St. Martin, a Canadian working for the American Fur Company at Fort Mackinac, Michigan, was wounded by a shotgun blast in 1822. Dr. Beaumont, the treating physician, saved Martin's life; however, the patient's wound never healed completely, and he was left with an exterior hole that led to his stomach. A piece of flesh covered the opening, which allowed Dr. Beaumont to view the stomach and to extract and analyze gastric juices along with Martin's stomach contents at various stages of digestion. His research showed that stomach acid, not just the mashing and squeezing of stomach contents, was an essential component of digestion. It was no longer just a mechanical process but a chemical process as well. This early research formed the basis of our modern knowledge of digestion.[2]

When you take a bite of food and begin chewing, salivary glands release saliva, which contains amylase. Amylase is an enzyme that aids in the digestion of starch. When you swallow, the food enters the pharynx, and an automatic involuntary reflex takes over that causes the epiglottis (leaf-shaped structure located immediately behind the root of the tongue) to cover the entrance to the larynx (voice box). This prevents food or liquids from entering the airway and traveling to your lungs instead of your stomach.

As you swallow, the food goes down your throat and heads toward a sphincter (ring of muscle) at the top of the esophagus. The esophagus responds to the food by relaxing, thus allowing the food to enter the stomach.

The stomach continues digestion by mixing the chewed food with digestive juices and utilizing the muscles of the stomach. The three layers of stomach muscle are made up of circular, diagonal, and longitudinal layers. They churn and squeeze the stomach contents. The stomach is capable of holding under two quarts of semidigested food. This semidigested food stays in the stomach for approximately three to five hours. That is why it is recommended that you space out your meals at five-hour intervals (more on that in chapter 7), giving the stomach a chance to digest what you have eaten without being bombarded with another dump of food. Although the stomach works on digesting food, it is unable to absorb food; however, it can absorb alcohol. This explains why alcohol can have a stronger effect, along with a rapid impact, when you drink on an "empty" stomach, right?

The churning action of the stomach breaks up solid semidigested food into smaller particles. Chemical changes also occur due to enzymes in the gastric juices. The partially digested food then leaves the stomach and continues to the small intestine, where it is broken down into fats, proteins, and carbohydrates, including glucose (the metabolized form of sugar), and mixed with more digestive juices from the small intestine, pancreas, and liver. Important digestive enzymes from the pancreas and liver are released through ducts into the small intestine. At this point, digestion becomes interesting. What you have eaten can be either good or bad for your pancreas, your weight, and your health.

Take your right hand, touch your thumb to your baby finger, and place the rest of your hand (pointer, middle, and ring fingers) facing left just below your sternum (breastbone). This is where your pancreas lies, right behind your stomach and your baby finger along with your thumb is where your pancreas connects with the small intestine.

The pancreas secretes hormones and enzymes into the blood (endocrine function) or into the gastrointestinal tract (exocrine function). The pancreas's endocrine job is to produce insulin and glucagon. These hormones are released in response to meals and regulate glucose levels in the blood. Insulin is required to transfer molecules of glucose from the blood into cells throughout the body. Insulin acts like a key that opens the cell's door for glucose/fuel to enter. Without it, glucose will not be able to get inside any cells.

Glucagon, however, is a hormone that raises the level of glucose in the blood. Our bodies evolved to compensate for our historically inconsistent food supply. We have storage tanks for extra fuel in case there is no food. In the time of early humanity, periods of famine were common. Today, even with an oversaturation of food, you may not have eaten because you were too busy: you had a full day of meetings, business travel, or parenting children, or maybe you did a strenuous workout that required more fuel. Whatever the case may be, your cells still need a steady supply of glucose to function, so the pancreas releases glucagon, which stimulates the liver and muscles to release glucose from glycogen.

The pancreas's exocrine function is to produce digestive enzymes and bicarbonate. Both bicarbonate and insulin are released into the lumen of the small intestine by way of the pancreatic duct. (Remember when I asked you to touch your thumb to your baby finger and place your hand below your sternum? The visual is important.) Since the stomach produces an intensely acidic environment, food moving from the stomach to the small intestine needs to be neutralized. Bicarbonate works to create a neutral pH, which protects the intestine from acid damage while establishing an environment that allows other pancreatic enzymes to do their thing. These enzymes assist in the further breakdown of food into small molecules that can be transferred into the bloodstream and processed by cells.

After all the nutrients are absorbed through the small intestinal walls and transported throughout the body via the bloodstream, the resulting waste material, including fiber and old cells, is pushed into the large intestine, where it remains until expelled in a bowel movement.[3]

Keep in mind that the body's principal source of energy is glucose. From the small intestine, it crosses the intestinal membrane and is absorbed into the bloodstream. Glucose is then carried through the bloodstream and either used by the cells of the body or stored. Too much glucose is unhealthy.

In response to high levels of glucose in the bloodstream, the pancreas produces and releases insulin. If you eat the wrong foods, eat large portions, combine foods improperly (we'll get to this topic in chapter 14), and/or lead a sedentary lifestyle, then, instead of being used, the food/glucose/fuel is stored. It is stored in the form of glycogen in the liver and muscles (for emergency fuel) and as fat in the rest of the body. Too much glucose becomes ineffective, useless fuel, and weight gain will reflect that. Unfortunately, obesity produces a vicious cycle by impairing the body's responsiveness to insulin. The more weight you carry, the more your body is unresponsive to the insulin "key," which in turn raises blood sugar and insulin levels and increases weight gain.

When the insulin key is unable to unlock the cell door, rendering it ineffective, this situation is referred to as insulin resistance. When this happens, the excess glucose and insulin course through your bloodstream until they are eventually excreted or stored. This situation is highly inflammatory to your blood vessels, your kidneys, and your entire body.

Food has an effect on every organ and every cell in your body. If you abuse your pancreas with the wrong food, your blood glucose rises and your pancreas responds accordingly. Glucagon likewise signals the liver to secrete not just glucose but also triglycerides (rich lipid particles). Those particles are released into your bloodstream when the liver reaches its storage capacity. If you see high triglyceride numbers, think about insulin and glucose and their effect on heart disease.

So please think before you eat anything. Ask yourself whether what you are about to put in your mouth is a good or bad choice of fuel for your body. As the saying goes, "You are what you eat." Remember, it begins with your mouth, and every choice has an effect on every part of your organic machine, from your weight to your heart. Every cell and tissue of your body is alive and should be treated with the utmost respect, never abused. Your entire digestive system is not made of steel or rubber. It is organic, and it does its best every day to deal with your choices—what you decide to eat and drink and whether you choose to exercise.

The next time you think about ordering that bacon burger with fries and washing it down with a soda, please think about how each bite will affect your entire digestive system and whether it is the healthiest fuel to properly operate your body, provide well-being, and ensure a healthy weight.

Remember my mantra and imprint it in your brain: Your mouth is NOT supposed to have a party at every meal!

How Do High Glucose and Insulin Affect Weight and Health?

"Life is really simple, but we insist
on making it complicated."

—CONFUCIUS

I believe the pancreas is the gatekeeper of good health versus poor health, weight gain versus weight loss. When unwise food and beverage choices affect your blood glucose and insulin levels, you can expect weight gain and poor health. Let me give you a basic understanding of how noncommunicable diseases (NCDs) are a result of unhealthy glucose and insulin levels.

Heart disease (high blood pressure, high cholesterol, and atherosclerosis) is a result of excess glucose and high insulin levels. High levels of glucose due to unwise food choices, obesity, and stress lead to high levels of insulin, which are inflammatory and extremely toxic to the lining of your veins, arteries, and capillaries.

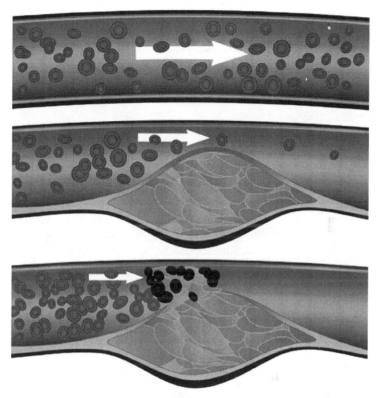

High levels of glucose and insulin = inflammation =
cardiovascular disease.

Source: © iStock/Getty Images Plus/Diamond_Images

This chronic inflammation can cause "sores" in the lining of
your veins, arteries, and capillaries. Because your body is hardwired to heal itself, it will attempt to heal that sore, and an internal "scab" can form. The scab acts as a "speed bump" where bad
fats can collect, narrowing the diameter of your vessels. Atherosclerosis refers to the buildup of fats, cholesterol, and other substances in your arteries and on your artery walls (plaque), which
can restrict blood flow. In addition, the chronic inflammation
creates a further narrowing of the vessels due to swelling. This

narrowing makes it more difficult for the heart to pump blood through your vessels (think of stepping on a water hose), resulting in high blood pressure.

If by chance a fat particle or blood clot takes off in your circulatory system, you are in for a heart attack, stroke, or pulmonary embolism. Chronic inflammation and cholesterol levels can be responsible.

Total cholesterol numbers showcase the amount of cholesterol (a waxy, fat-like substance found in every cell of your body) by including LDL (low-density lipoprotein; "bad cholesterol"), HDL (high-density lipoprotein; "good" cholesterol), and triglycerides (fats).

Triglycerides help transport cholesterol—which is essential for brain and nerve function—to your cells. They also carry glucose, or blood sugar, to your fat cells. I'm sure you already know that triglycerides are found in foods such as butter and oil, but you might not know that your body also makes triglycerides from excess calories, especially from alcohol and simple carbohydrates found in sugar-rich foods.

Increased glucose leads to excess body fat, which raises levels of LDL and triglycerides. This situation contributes to lower HDL levels. High triglycerides coupled with high LDL levels elevate your chance of having a heart attack. High levels of triglycerides increase your risk not only for heart disease but also for liver disease.

It's true, insulin signals the liver to secrete excess nutrients (glucose) into triglyceride-rich lipid particles. Those particles are released into your bloodstream when the liver reaches its capacity. A liver that has to deal with constantly being "full" is going to become "sick." A full, fatty liver is as often caused by high glucose levels as by high fat levels.

So, if you see unhealthy cholesterol numbers, please think about insulin and glucose. Your body is speaking to you. Address the root cause and do not expect medication (statin drugs) to relieve you of your *self-health responsibility*.

Cholesterol Guidelines

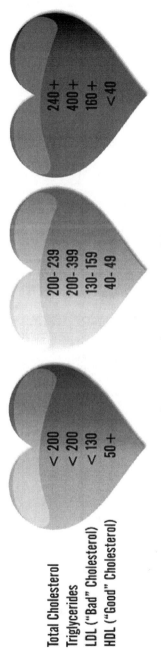

Total Cholesterol	< 200	200-239	240 +
Triglycerides	< 200	200-399	400 +
LDL ("Bad" Cholesterol)	< 130	130-159	160 +
HDL ("Good" Cholesterol)	50 +	40-49	< 40

What category do your numbers fall into without a statin medication?

Source: Natalie Rosen

The following NCDs are explained in basic terms and are often linked to high cholesterol, triglycerides, glucose, and insulin:

High cholesterol is a result of high fat, glucose, and insulin levels.

High blood pressure is a result of the narrowing of the blood vessels, which are inflamed due to increased insulin levels and/or fatty deposits (see above for the full explanation).

Polycystic ovarian syndrome (in women) is the result of high insulin levels that reduce the production of estrogen by the ovaries, which results in increased levels of androgens (testosterone). It is associated with unwanted facial hair, weight gain, irregular periods, acne, infertility, and eventually heart disease and diabetes; it can also increase your incidence of cancer.

Low testosterone (in men) may be the result of high insulin levels that reduce the production of testosterone and cause a rise in estrogen levels. This leads to sexual dysfunction, impotence (the need for Viagra), "man boobs," and reduced facial hair. Men, a word of advice: change your diet, and you'll change your manhood!

Insulin resistance is a condition in which cells (particularly those of muscle, fat, and liver tissue) display "resistance" to insulin by failing to take up and utilize glucose for energy and metabolism. The pancreas responds to the resulting increased glucose levels in the bloodstream by producing more insulin.

Metabolic syndrome is a result of high glucose and high insulin. Excess and unused "fuel" is often stored as "belly" fat.

Renal disease occurs when high levels of glucose and insulin damage the kidneys' sophisticated filtration system. This inflames the kidneys, whose job is to filter and flush food and beverage choices out of your body. Constantly filtering toxins has a cumulative effect on your poor kidneys.

Type 2 diabetes occurs when high levels of glucose demand that your pancreas secrete large amounts of insulin. This takes a toll on your poor pancreas, which cannot keep up with the demands imposed by unwise choices. The insulin key is rendered ineffective, and eventually the pancreas burns out.

I'd like to emphasize how important it is for parents to be vigilant about their children's nutrition if they want to prevent type 2 diabetes. The way a parent shops, cooks, and eats has a direct impact on a child's health. Proper nutrition, along with activity rather than inactivity, is crucial to preventing obesity and type 2 diabetes.

Childhood obesity is out of control: 41 million children under the age of five and over 340 million children and adolescents aged five to nineteen were overweight or obese in 2016.[1] This is disgraceful! Obesity has led to a dramatic increase in the incidence of type 2 diabetes among children and adolescents over the past two decades.

Years ago the majority of diabetes cases among children and adolescents were immune-mediated diabetes, referred to as type 1 diabetes. Type 2 diabetes was commonly referred to as "adult-onset diabetes," only affecting middle-aged adults. Well, not anymore. Type 2 diabetes is now diagnosed in five- and eight-year-olds.

Obesity is strongly associated with insulin resistance (remember the insulin key and how it is rendered ineffective?), which leads to the development of type 2 diabetes. The tragedy of a type 2 diabetes diagnosis in children and adolescents is the offshoot diseases they may experience earlier in life as a result.

Typically these offshoot diseases occur anywhere from two to twenty years after a diabetes diagnosis in adults, depending on how vigilant patients are about controlling their blood glucose, which is also reflected in the corresponding biomarker hemoglobin A1c levels. So if you are diagnosed with type 2 diabetes at the age of forty-five, then you might not experience eye, kidney, nerve, or heart disease until you are in your sixties. Now think about an eight-year-old diagnosed with type 2 diabetes. What will his or her health future look like in twenty years at the age of twenty-eight?

I think it is parents' responsibility to feed their children correctly. Your food choices have a direct effect on your children's present and future health and well-being. Remember, obesity is preventable, and so is type 2 diabetes!

And let's not forget cancer. Potential cancerous cells reside within each and every one of our bodies. For most of us, they remain dormant, but for others, a switch is turned on. Genetics, toxic environmental factors, smoking, radiation, medication (e.g., hormone-replacement therapy and birth control pills), and obesity can all determine whether that switch is flipped. Contrary to popular belief, only between 5 and 10 percent of cancers are caused solely by genetic risk (according to the National Cancer Institute), and as I stated earlier, obesity has replaced tobacco use as the leading preventable cause of cancer.[2]

Eating to reverse NCDs is extraordinarily important and life saving. Eating to *prevent* a disease is crucial. Why would anyone want to deal with a health issue that is preventable? Data-Driven Fueling will enable you to help you maintain healthy glucose and insulin levels that will ultimately benefit not just you but also your loved ones.

Hormones, Stress, and Weight

Several hormones, including cortisol, leptin, insulin, and sex hormones, have been studied extensively for their role in obesity and body weight. These hormones play a role in appetite, metabolism, body-fat distribution, and increased storage of excess energy from food as fats. Obese people have levels of these hormones that can increase accumulation of body fat by altering the metabolism of their fat cells.

Cortisol

The "stress hormone" cortisol helps us survive short periods of stress (whether due to an emotional issue, an infection, or another health problem). Cortisol benefits the body during short bouts of stress by increasing blood sugar (causing the muscles and the liver to release glycogen into the bloodstream), fuel for immediate energy, increasing immune response, decreasing the body's response to pain, enhancing short-term memory, and extracting calcium from our bones to be utilized by muscles for quick action.

Although cortisol's mission is to aid the body in recovering from acute stressful situations, chronically increased cortisol levels are detrimental to the body. Unfortunately, in today's society, the human body and mind endure long periods of chronic stress, which lead to chronically elevated levels of cortisol.

High levels of cortisol compromise the immune system and increase blood pressure and blood glucose. The pancreas responds to the increased blood glucose by producing and secreting more insulin. This state of hyperinsulinemia (excess insulin) is toxic to the organs and vessels of the body. This situation places the body in a highly inflammatory state, which is totally unhealthy.

So, how is cortisol connected to the stress response?

The adrenal glands are small, triangular-shaped endocrine (hormone-producing) glands located on top of each kidney. These glands produce several hormones when we perceive ourselves to be in a dangerous situation. The most important, adrenaline (think "fight or flight") and cortisol, are regulated by the nervous and immune systems and secreted into the bloodstream. When the adrenal glands are called into action, they produce a "rush of adrenaline," as well as a release of the "stress hormone" cortisol.

Beyond the appearance of the occasional saber-toothed tiger, the fight-or-flight response was not a regular occurrence for our ancestors. However, these days, fast-paced living, decreased sleep, unemployment, stress in the workplace, financial insecurity, violence, fear for personal safety, poor nutrition, limited exercise, and obesity—not to mention environmental toxins—all have an effect on the fight-or-flight response. Once cortisol is released, it lingers in your body for approximately two hours. This leads to chronically elevated levels, much like a constant intravenous drip of cortisol. This constant drip impedes weight loss and adversely affects your health. That is why stress-reduction techniques are so important and must be incorporated into your daily life. Stress-reduction options are listed at the end of this chapter.

Leptin

Leptin is a hormone manufactured in adipose (fat) cells. It helps regulate energy balance by inhibiting hunger, but it can also affect weight gain.

When leptin is released in amounts *proportional* to normal body weight, it reaches the brain and binds with its receptors. This process informs the body that it has reached its capacity. Because leptin is produced by fat cells, leptin levels tend to be higher in obese people than in people with a healthier weight/height proportion.

Some overweight people may wonder, *Well, if my body makes more leptin because I'm fat, then I should have zero appetite, right?* Unfortunately, the opposite appears to be the case. Overweight people never feel full or satisfied. Sadly, with obesity also comes a resistance to leptin's effect. Those high levels are wasted because your brain isn't getting the message. In laymen's terms, the brain hasn't heard that you just ate dinner; it thinks that you haven't eaten or that you haven't eaten enough.

This situation is referred to as leptin insensitivity/resistance. It appears to be linked to a deficiency in leptin receptors. Some scientists believe that this phenomenon is linked to insulin resistance and the associated hyperinsulinemia. Remember, I believe the pancreas is the gatekeeper of good health versus poor health and weight gain versus weight loss.

This inability of insulin or leptin to initiate a healthy response drives the production of more insulin and more weight gain. Imagine a cell in your body impeding the uptake of glucose by saying, "I'm full." This situation only drives the pancreas to produce more insulin, creating a vicious cycle—a cycle that can be broken as you Forget Dieting! and embrace the Data-Driven Fueling Lifestyle.

Insulin and Sex Hormones

The added excess insulin production by the pancreas results in hyperinsulinemia (too much insulin in your bloodstream).

Hyperinsulinemia interferes with your body's sex hormone balance. In women, high insulin levels reduce the production of estrogen, causing a rise in androgens (i.e., testosterone). By the same token, high insulin levels reduce the production of testosterone in men, causing a rise in estrogen. I refer to this condition in both men and women as *Adrenobesity*™.

Adrenobesity isn't just about food choices and portion control; it also has to do with the role stress plays in hormonal imbalance and ultimately weight gain. Stressors cause your body to produce and release inappropriate and/or increased amounts of adrenaline and cortisol.

Stress increases the dump of glucose and the overproduction of insulin, which causes your body to incorrectly process its fuel and leads to fat storage in your face, neck, arms, belly, butt, and thighs. This effect is compounded as we age. The main site for estrogen production in middle-aged men and postmenopausal women is fat cells. Therefore, excess fat cells impact the balance of testosterone and estrogen, which compromises the effectiveness of insulin. The result is weight gain and a "unisex" appearance. Men and women appear to have similar body shapes. This is not meant to offend. It is meant to illustrate the situation many find themselves in with no idea how they got there.

I believe most individuals who experience weight gain, poor health, and what I call Adrenobesity are truly victims. They are victims of misinformation, greedy food corporations, marketing gurus, and the inability of their health-care providers to spend quality time with them. However, once you are educated about your body and how food choices affect it, you are no longer a victim. The power resides in you.

Too many people have undergone a metamorphosis due to hormonal imbalance. Many men and women wonder what is behind the transformation, why their bodies have come to lack definition. Torsos (from the shoulders to the hips) are barrel shaped, arms and legs are puffy (like pincushions), and double or triple chins appear. The fat around the abdomen, a symptom of "metabolic syndrome," is linked to an increased risk of heart disease and other health conditions.

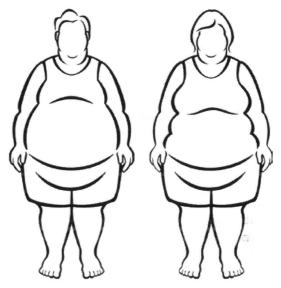

Increased insulin production due to increased glucose alters hormones, redistributes fat, and leads to a unisex appearance.

Source: © iStock/Getty Images Plus/kellykellykelly

Massive abdomens and "man boobs" embarrass many men.
Purchasing XXXL shirts is nothing they are proud of; yet they
have no idea how to tackle their expanding torsos. Besides man
boobs, some men and adolescent boys experience a decrease
in hair growth (little hair on their arms, legs, and chest, along
with an inability to grow a moustache or beard) and even erectile
dysfunction.

Obesity lowers the level of testosterone, the major male
hormone in teenage boys and men. A 2008 study of 1,862 men
(ages thirty and over) found that waist circumference was an
even stronger predictor of low testosterone levels than body mass
index. A four-inch increase in waist size increased a man's odds of
having a low testosterone level by 75 percent![1]

Women are also prone to barrel-shaped torsos, and their breasts
become part of their abdominal circumference. Some reason that
this is part of the aging process and menopause. It is not!

Obesity and pancreatic abuse alter the metabolism of sex hormones. Adult men and women are not the only ones dealing with Adrenobesity; girls and boys are also developing the same unisex look. It's not fair, and it is extremely unhealthy!!

None of this is normal. These physical manifestations are the only way the body can communicate with you. The body is screaming, "Help me!" Unfortunately, the cries for help are ignored because we don't understand that if we work with our bodies, they will respond in a positive way. There is a disassociation that needs to be corrected.

It's no secret that obesity is a big problem in the United States. Over two-thirds of all adult Americans need to lose weight, and the number of obese children is growing at a frightening rate. An overweight adolescent has a 70 percent chance of becoming an overweight or obese adult. Yes, this is due to eating the wrong foods, the wrong combination of foods, and pancreatic abuse, but Adrenobesity's main culprit is stress. Children are experiencing more stress than ever before. The number of children with diagnosed anxiety, not depression, has increased in recent years.[2]

The good news is that Adrenobesity is reversible. Knowledge about how food and stress affect you and your children will help you combat the problem effectively by addressing the root cause of stress and applying stress-relieving techniques.

Stress

Stress plays a significant role in weight gain. Stress increases not only your heart rate and blood pressure but also your blood glucose. The obesity epidemic is about more than food choices, activity, and portion control. It's also about stress. Traumatic events such as death or divorce can cause acute stress that has a dramatic impact on appetite. Even welcome and intentional events can cause stress. Human beings crave predictability and comfort. Change brings discomfort and anxiety. Also, fear of the unknown can fuel chronic stress. All of this affects our ability to lose weight and taxes our health.

One of my clients experienced a relaxing morning. Upon rising, her morning blood glucose was 78 mg/dL (well within the normal range of 70 mg/dL to 100 mg/dL; more on this in chapter 5), and ninety minutes after breakfast, it was 92 mg/dL. While driving to work, however, she was pulled over by a policeman for speeding. She became extremely upset, especially when the policeman issued a ticket. She sat in her car shaking. Remembering what I had told her about stress and its effect on blood glucose and weight, she took this opportunity to test my statement. She pulled her glucometer out of her purse, pricked her finger, and there it was: her blood glucose had spiked to 157 mg/dL!

Our lives are filled with uncertainty and instability. Interpersonal relationship issues, job troubles, health issues, financial struggles, and even a traffic ticket can impact our day-to-day lives. This effect is only compounded by the constant bombardment of doom-and-gloom news.

Additional, rarely addressed stressors are exercise and dieting. Carving out exercise time in a day causes stress. If you don't like the activity, you don't feel you are doing the yoga pose as well as the person next to you, or your exercise results are less than you hoped for, you can get stressed.

Dieting is stressful. Adhering to a specific diet, figuring out where to eat, or shopping for and preparing food all add to your day-to-day stress and are counterproductive to weight loss.

Forget Dieting! is not a diet. Once you accept that you are fueling instead of dieting and that you have embarked on a lifestyle of eating to protect your pancreas, your health, and your weight, you'll be a lot less stressed.

Realizing what you do and don't have control of is the first step in dealing with stress. The one thing I know for sure is that you have control over the following: what you put in your mouth, how much movement you do, and how you deal with stress.

How does stress affect weight and health? Your body is hardwired to respond to a perceived threat or demand by calling on the adrenal glands to release a flood of stress hormones.

Again, as I stated in the beginning of this chapter, while some hormones released during stress prepare the body for an emergency by making stored energy available, other hormones help the body store energy as fat, which facilitates weight gain.

When a fight-or-flight response isn't met with fighting or running away, you are left with a toxic situation for your body. When the adrenal glands release adrenaline and/or cortisol, you think less and react instinctively. Typically, the "crisis" is over in a matter of seconds or minutes, and your body chemistry and physical sensations return to normal. However, if you remain in a constant state of anxiety (ruminating about a problem at work or a financial issue, worrying about your personal health or that of a loved one, or even stressing out about exercise), then your adrenal glands will respond with a continuous drip of cortisol. This constant drip causes your body to incorrectly process food and store fat unnecessarily.

Stress can also lead to weight loss. Sudden weight loss is usually the result of a stressful event (changing jobs, divorce, or death); however, it can also be a sign of a serious illness (it is wise to report any sudden weight loss to your physician). The weight loss during stress is attributed to poor food choices (a bag of chips instead of lunch), missed meals, or a loss of appetite. The weight loss is often only temporary, and your weight will return to normal once you have recovered from the stressful event.

I know from experience. When my mother died, I was stressed and depressed. I had no appetite, and I lost weight. As the months passed, the pain of losing my mother gave way to a different stressor: caring for my widowed father. He had been completely dependent on my mother, and her death affected him on many levels. I dealt with that stress by self-soothing with food. So I gained back the weight I lost during the grieving process (and then some). Stress has an impact on weight gain.

The excessive release of glucose and the overproduction of insulin by constant stress creates an inflammatory state that makes losing weight difficult, even if you are watching every calorie. Remember, insulin acts as a key, unlocking your cells for glucose entry. But if your cells are already full because you are not actually burning glucose by fighting or running, the insulin is rendered ineffective, and the excess glucose is sent to fat cells for storage. Not good!

What Can You Do to Reduce the Effects of Stress on Your Weight and Health?

Get enough sleep (at least eight hours every night).

Eat to protect your pancreas by keeping your glucose between 70 and 100 mg/dL ninety minutes after you eat a meal or snack (this is covered in chapter 5).

Practice deep breathing. Inhale through your nose (to the count of 1, 2, 3, 4), hold your breath (1, 2, 3, 4), and then exhale (4, 3, 2, 1). Do this in the morning when you wake up and again several times a day. You can practice this breathing technique by doing it every time you get a text message (breathe before looking at it), every time you arrive at a stop sign or stoplight, or before you get in your car or on a bus or train. Before you know it, deep breathing will become part of your muscle memory and your go-to coping mechanism when stressed. Remember to fill your lung buckets completely, not just a quarter or half full. Inhale as if you are filling up your entire abdomen too. Abdominal breathing reduces anxiety and stress. As you incorporate deep breathing into your daily routine, you increase the supply of oxygen to your brain, which stimulates the parasympathetic nervous system (slowing down the heart rate and relaxing muscles), creating a state of calm. By becoming more connected to your body, you get out of your head, quieting the chatty, negative thoughts running through your mind.

Take a hot bath.

Get a massage. You don't need to go to a massage therapist. You can take lotion and massage your own hands and feet.

Use essential oils, like lavender, rose, or vetiver on your pillow or in your bath. I've tried all three separately and find that they do provide a calming effect.

Increase your activity. Movement/exercise soothes the mind by releasing endorphins. Take a walk around your neighborhood or in a park. Take notice of sounds and sights. Listen to the bird chatter; observe flowers, trees, and other vegetation. Before you know it, you've walked thirty minutes. Increased activity (especially important for children) forces your body to go into your "storage tanks/fat cells" for fuel to operate your living machine (see chapter 10 on movement).

Practice meditation. Set aside ten minutes a day (twice a day would be even better) to tune in to yourself and release your mind from chatty thoughts.

Listen to music, watch a video, or look at a photograph. These also work for me. I will listen to Bobby McFerrin's "Don't Worry, Be Happy," look at photos of my granddaughter, or watch videos on my phone of my horses. Find your "something" that takes you out of the moment and brings a smile to your face.

Spend time with your pet. Animals love you unconditionally. You can tell them anything and know that none of it will be repeated!

Light a scented candle. Just like essentials oils, certain scents can have a calming effect and lift your spirits.

Avoid too much caffeine and/or alcohol and too many energy drinks. Too much caffeine can actually increase feelings of anxiety. This includes illegal substances.

Seek counseling. A therapist can help you identify stressors in your life and provide coping tools for your specific situation.

Evaluate each stressful situation. Can you control it? Write down the stressful situation in your journal—journaling is critical to self-reflection and behavior modification and is covered in chapter 17—and then brainstorm realistic solutions. Some things are just out of our hands. Know the difference between what you can control and what you cannot.

Incorporate this motto into your thinking: "It is what it is!" If you can't control it, just let go. I know this is difficult to do, but it is part of your transformation, your behavior modification. I've gotten myself into stressful states ruminating about situations and have learned repeatedly that all that cortisol and adrenaline that raised my blood pressure had no effect on the situation. The only effect was on my body and my health. So what do I do? I deep breathe; I meditate; I go on YouTube, select a meditative, calming piece, and set the timer on my phone for ten minutes during which I do not allow any chatty thoughts to enter my mind. It's a ten-minute break from stress. Any time a chatty thought creeps in, I acknowledge it, release it, and focus on the music.

Remember that beating your head against a wall makes it difficult to solve even the simplest problem. Getting yourself into a tizzy works against clear thinking and impedes your ability to solve a problem or issue. It is also important to embrace patience and realize that many issues will work themselves out over time without your doing anything.

Armed with this information and an understanding of chronic stress and its impact on weight gain, it is up to you to break the cycle with stress reducers. You can jump-start your new lifestyle of improved health and weight loss through effective management of stress, movement, and data-driven fueling.

Remember, weight loss occurs when you take in the correct food/fuel for your body, maintain a consistent blood sugar between 70 and 100 mg/dL, increase your activity, and reduce and control stress. Only when you actively participate in the practice of self-health will weight loss, improved health, and well-being occur.

Section II

Data-Driven Fueling

"A wise man should consider that health
is the greatest of human blessings."

—HIPPOCRATES

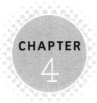

Data-Driven Fueling Guidelines

> "The best way of learning about
> anything is by doing."
>
> —RICHARD BRANSON

Your thought process about losing weight has to change from dieting to fueling.

Revolutionize yourself through Data-Driven Fueling (DDF), the self-health approach to sustainable weight loss and improved health and well-being. Forget Dieting! You are armed with information about how to properly care for yourself and how food affects your body; why would you ever need to diet again?

The Basic Principles of Data-Driven Fueling

#1: *Your Mouth Is Not Supposed to Have a Party at Every Meal*

Remember that food is fuel. You eat to sustain life, not destroy it. You can enjoy food, but eating as if every meal is your last will damage your health and could even become a self-fulfilling prophecy. Keep this image in mind: your body is a finely calibrated organic machine, not some inorganic waste receptacle.

#2: Less Is More

You don't need to give in to the breakfast buffet. Order an egg-white omelet with veggies and a small side salad off the menu. It's cheaper than the buffet and better for you. You don't have to clean your plate, either. Leave at least one forkful of food on your plate, or eat half and take the leftovers for tomorrow's lunch.

#3: Move

Moving does not mean vigorous exercise. In fact, I've discovered that if you have over forty pounds to lose, low-impact activity (such as walking, yoga, or swimming) is actually more effective. Overly strenuous exercise when you have a lot to lose can have a negative effect on your joints and back. Additionally, I believe that building muscle when you have a significant amount of weight to lose only compresses the adipose (fat) tissue between your muscles and your skin, making it harder to shed. Once you have lost a substantial amount of weight (again, if you have over forty pounds to lose), you can sculpt and define your body with appropriate, potentially more strenuous movement and weights. It's most important that you move your body, get your blood circulating, and use your fuel! A sedentary lifestyle is an unhealthy lifestyle (see chapter 10 for more information about movement/exercise).

#4: Test or "Tune In" to Protect Your Pancreas

The goal is to maintain a blood sugar/glucose level between 70 and 100 mg/dL ninety minutes after you eat a meal or a snack to avoid an insulin surge from your pancreas. In order to do this, you will have to test your blood with a glucometer (a needle prick) as a diabetic does. There are new devices on the market: Dexcom and Libre

Pro utilize a disc placed on your upper arm that is replaced every two weeks. Whatever device you decide on will be used for two to three months or until you get an understanding of what your organic machine feels is healthy or unhealthy for you. If you tune in, your focus will be on the assessment of bodily feelings rather than glucometer readings. You'll learn how to do this in chapter 5.

#5: Listen to Your Body

If you have to take a deep breath or unbutton your pants before your next bite, your body is telling you that it is full! Listen up! Put down your fork and knife, push your plate away, and get up from the table.

#6: Remove Unhealthy Temptations

Please don't force your mind into a dilemma of unhealthy choices: eliminate temptation at home and at work. If ice cream in the refrigerator poses a temptation, pitch it. If potato chips, cheese, and crackers are your go-to snack, don't buy them! Dump the cookies in your desk drawer at work and pretend the junk food vending machine at the end of the hall doesn't exist. Temptations in your environment make healthy eating much more difficult. Figure out a way to eliminate temptations that trigger poor choices.

What to Avoid

> Anything white (white flour bread, white flour pasta, white potatoes, white rice, white sugar)
>
> Dairy (cheese, yogurt, milk, ice cream)
>
> Sweets (donuts, cakes, cookies)
>
> Sugars (artificial and regular)
>
> Sodas (diet or regular)
>
> Any foods you see advertised on television

Eating fruit with other foods (there are two exceptions—refer to chapter 14)

Cooked corn and cooked carrots

Processed foods

Improper food combinations

Stress

A sedentary lifestyle

You wouldn't pour a milkshake into your car's gas tank or fill it with so much gas that it overflowed, would you? How about feeding your dog chocolate? You must be mindful about what you put in your mouth. If you know certain foods are unhealthy, even harmful, why would you eat them?

The DDF guidelines provide the framework for your DDF lifestyle. Your body is a miraculous, organic, vital machine that deserves the utmost care. Your lungs never forget to take a breath. Your heart beats with precise regularity. Your organic machine is not a garbage can for you to pollute with junk foods or the wrong food combinations. If you treat it like a garbage can, then you should expect the consequences.

However, if you respect your machine and provide it with the necessary tools (nourishment, movement/exercise, and stress reduction), it will do its best to promote health and achieve an appropriate weight. It wants to work with you because every minute of every day it is focused on survival, keeping you alive. The following chapters will help you understand your machine and what you can do to help yourself. Are you up for the challenge to change and *Forget Dieting!*?

CHAPTER 5

The Data-Driven
Fueling Lifestyle

Disclaimer: Before you begin any new diet and/or exercise program, you must inform your physician, especially if you are on medication. The Data-Driven Fueling lifestyle may reduce or eliminate your need for medication. If you are a type 1 or type 2 diabetic on insulin, your units may need to be altered. You don't want to place yourself in a position of hypoglycemia (low blood sugar). If you are on high blood pressure medication, your blood pressure may change as you change your diet. Be vigilant about taking your blood pressure. Do not place yourself in a compromised position of low blood pressure. It is critical that you make sure your physician is aware. You are in a partnership with your physician and communication is critical. He or she may need to alter your medication.

When you inform your physician that you have started the Data-Driven Fueling program, please request blood work (full chemistry panel including fasting blood glucose) before beginning DDF. It will provide a baseline of information. Repeat the blood work after four months of Data-Driven Fueling. This information adds to the data you will collect over the four-month process of changing your eating habits. In addition, it is important to take measurements of your chest, waist, hips, upper arms, and thighs before beginning DDF and then every four months until your one-year DDF anniversary. The accumulated data will showcase your transformation and serve as the major reason you have decided to Forget Dieting! and fuel instead.

> "When I let go of what I am,
> I become what I might be."
>
> —LAO TZU

M y guess is you decided to buy this book because you are sick and tired of diets. In fact, you *hate* even the idea of dieting. Data-Driven Fueling is a lifelong plan to help you help yourself. The cornerstone of DDF lies in your acceptance of it as your lifestyle and not another diet. This is your new norm and the way you are going to eat for the rest of your life if you want to maintain health and sustain weight loss.

There are thousands of diets out there. On January 2, 2019, *U.S. News & World Report* listed the top forty-one best diets overall.[1] With so many to choose from, I am often asked what sets my program apart from all the others.

Data-Driven Fueling is a lifestyle based on hard-core data if you choose to test with a glucometer. It is not an eating plan to drop a quick twenty pounds. It is about fueling, not dieting. It offers sustainable weight loss and improved health and well-being based on precision nutrition.

Your body is a living organic machine (I can't emphasize this fact enough). Supplied with an understanding of how your body processes what you eat and how it communicates with you all day long (via sensations, thoughts, blood glucose readings, the mirror, and the scale), you cannot turn a blind eye or a deaf ear. Data-Driven Fueling takes the guesswork out of knowing what to feed yourself.

Keto, Paleo, Atkins, South Beach, and Dukan are some of the popular diets today. I have no problem with clients who go on these diets because they are in a rush and want to drop a quick five to ten pounds before a special event or beach vacation; however, diets that push high-fat or high-animal-protein intake are not healthy over the long term.

The goal of low-carb diets is to reach a state of ketosis in which the body uses fat rather than glucose as fuel. Ketosis forces the liver to produce ketones from stored fat. That may sound great, especially if you are carrying a lot of fat on your body frame, but there is a price to pay when you are just burning fat.

Your body is hardwired to survive and will create ketones if you don't have enough insulin (in the case of diabetes) or are restricting your carb intake. Remember, carbs are converted into glucose—that is, fuel for your body. So if your body doesn't have any glucose to burn from what you are eating, then it has to rely on another source: fat.

Ketones are a type of acid that the liver sends into your bloodstream to fuel your muscles and other tissues. For a person without diabetes, this process doesn't become an issue; however, if you have diabetes, you can build up too many ketones in your bloodstream, and that can become life threatening.

High-fat and high-protein diets can play havoc with your kidneys. The kidneys excrete proteins and their breakdown products (for example, urea). If your diet's focus is lots of protein, then you are overloading them. A high-protein diet may worsen kidney function if you have kidney disease because your body is already struggling to eliminate waste products in general and may have trouble eliminating all the additional waste products of protein metabolism. You are only asking for more problems if you add to their burden.[2] In addition, the liver is stressed producing ketones. If you have any liver issues, this will only make them worse.

The reduction of fruits, vegetables, and grains in high-fat and high-protein diets may put you at risk for vitamin deficiencies. Other side effects of these diets include bad breath, constipation, and issues with concentration and mood swings (the brain needs glucose to operate properly).

And let's not forget the heart. High-fat and high-animal-protein diets can raise cholesterol levels and thus be risky for heart patients.

Again, these diets might offer a good short-term/quick-fix solution, but I wouldn't recommend them for long-term, sustainable health and weight loss. Severely restrictive diets have significant side effects and are difficult to sustain. Once you resume a "normal" diet, the weight you've lost will most likely return.

The DDF program promotes the practice of self-health and protects the pancreas—the gatekeeper of good versus bad health, weight gain versus weight loss. Your objective is to accept change. You are going to have to change your thought process and in turn your behavior concerning food: the way you purchase, cook, and eat.

The results will have a profound impact on your body and free you from dieting. Data-Driven Fueling affords a peek into your bio-individuality by providing an opportunity for self-discovery. Your body will tell you ninety minutes after you finish a meal or a snack what food and beverages work for you. I know I sound like a broken record, but the goal is to keep your blood sugar between 70 and 100 mg/dL. What does mg/dL (milligrams per deciliter) mean? A milligram is one-thousandth of a gram. A gram is about one-thirtieth of an ounce. A deciliter is one-tenth of a liter. A liter is a bit bigger than a quart. When your blood is tested, the measurement showcases the amount of a substance (in this case, glucose) in a specific amount of blood.

The A1c test is used to diagnose and monitor type 1 and type 2 diabetics. Individuals are tested every three months. The A1c test measures how much of hemoglobin (a protein in red blood cells that carries oxygen) is coated with sugar/glucose. The higher the number, the more glucose the hemoglobin is dealing with (not good).

There are two ways to approach Data-Driven Fueling: (1) testing or (2) tuning in. Testing tells you exactly how much glucose is in your blood ninety minutes after you eat, while tuning in lets you use your feelings as an approximation. Whether you test or tune in, make sure you purchase a scale because you need to weigh yourself every morning. You are collecting data on your most important research project: you!

Before you begin Data-Driven Fueling, I want you to eat as you normally would for two to three days. Journal your activity, meals, glucose numbers or tuning-in sensations, stress level, and sleep. This will provide a baseline before you begin your new lifestyle.

Testing

If you decide to test, you will use a glucometer, a device used by diabetics to obtain blood glucose levels. You will test four to six times per day, depending on the number of meals or snacks you consume for approximately three to four months.

Equipment you will need to test: a glucometer, alcohol swabs, lancets (needles), test strips, and a journal. You do not need a prescription from a physician to purchase a glucometer. However,

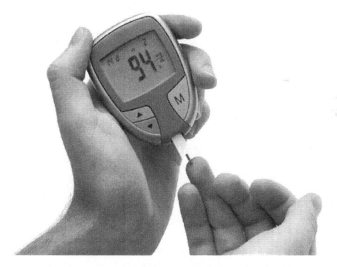

The glucometer provides accurate data that enables you to better understand how your organic machine processes what you eat—yet another way your body communicates with you.

Source: © iStock/Getty Images Plus/AlexRaths

prediabetics and diabetics can request a prescription from their physician to receive insurance coverage.

Various glucometers are available, such as the FreeStyle, OneTouch, Accu-Chek, Contour Next, and Fora Test N'Go.

You can buy your supplies at any pharmacy or online. A typical glucometer is relatively inexpensive, costing between $20 and $30. As with a printer, while the initial cost of the device is reasonable, the major expense is in the consumables (think ink cartridges). The glucometer expense is in the testing strips, which come in containers of fifty or one hundred. For example, Free-Style Lite strips cost between $20 and $35 for fifty. Buying in bulk, online, or during promotional sales will help reduce costs. Alcohol swabs and lancets are inexpensive. The good news is that you will only be testing for three to four months (the more vigilant you are about testing or tuning in, the sooner you will understand how food affects you). If your physician writes a prescription, then your insurance will cover the majority of the costs. In any case, investing in your health today will end up saving you money on health care in the future!

Two new devices on the market—Libre Pro and Dexcom—do not require finger pricks and are continuous glucose monitoring devices. Each is the size of a quarter and contains a small filament (needle) that when inserted lies just under the skin of your upper arm. Think of the device as a stamp. To apply it, you literally "stamp" it on your upper arm. It is self-adhesive and water resistant. I've applied this device to myself and my clients many times. It doesn't hurt.

You don't have to do anything. The sensor continuously measures your glucose via interstitial fluid (fluid found in spaces around cells that leak out of capillaries, small blood vessels), which provides you and your physician with important data on how your body reacts to food, beverages, stress, and movement. A small transmitter the size of a pager is scanned over the device on your arm and will provide a reading.

The device continually records blood glucose The Libre Pro and Dexcom require a physician's prescription and must be changed out every two weeks by you, a nurse, or a physician's assistant.

The cost is between $60 and $75 with insurance. One drawback to these continuous glucose monitoring devices versus traditional glucometers is that they may underreport glucose (40 percent of the time). Studies have shown that when the device indicated that user glucose values were at or below 60 mg/dL (hypoglycemia), user glucose values were actually in the range of 81 to 160 mg/dL. If you are a brittle diabetic, this would be of concern; however, for the purposes of weight loss and generalized improved health, these devices provide working data to aid in making necessary changes.

I have found with my clients and myself that the readings for the first twenty-four hours were inaccurate. The device apparently took that amount of time to adjust to the user's body chemistry. After twenty-four hours I noted that readings from the implanted device and a traditional glucometer differed by approximately five to ten points (the glucometer being more accurate). I suggest getting a baseline, which means (if you have a glucometer or you know someone who has one) using the glucometer to prick your finger and comparing that glucose result with that of the implanted device. If the glucometer reading is 81 mg/dL and the implanted device result is 75 mg/dL, then you'll know that the latter is six points off. Keep that in mind with all readings.

YouTube videos, health-care professionals, and pharmacists provide instruction on how to use the implant devices and any of the glucometers.

Testing requires you to check your blood ninety minutes after you finish a meal or a snack. Let's say you usually take fifteen to twenty minutes to eat breakfast. You would test ninety minutes after you finish (e.g., eat breakfast at 8:00 a.m., finish at 8:15, test at 9:45). If it took you thirty minutes to eat breakfast and you finished at 8:30 a.m., then test at 10:00 a.m. If two or more hours go by, just forget about testing after that meal. The results will be useless for your purposes. Wait until your next meal and test after that. Make sure to journal your results (see chapter 17 for more details about journaling).

Never allow your blood sugar to go below 70 mg/dL. When your blood sugar dips below 70 mg/dL, you can experience the symptoms of low blood sugar (lightheadedness, cravings, and even fainting). I know my limits. My blood sugar can go as low as 65 mg/dL before I begin to have symptoms of hypoglycemia. I am careful never to go below 65.

Interpreting the data is very important in your Forget Dieting! approach to living. As I stated, the goal is to keep your blood glucose between 70 and 100 mg/dL ninety minutes after you eat; however, you need to be aware of numerical spreads. Let's say you wake up, test your blood, and your reading is 72 mg/dL. Ninety minutes after breakfast, you test, and your glucose is now 104 mg/dL. You might think that 104 mg/dL is close enough to 100 mg/dL, so you would assume that breakfast was a good choice. Wrong. A spike of thirty-plus points is too much. Rethink what you ate. Is there something you could add to or omit from that breakfast choice to reduce the glucose spike? A spread of thirty-plus means that what you ate wasn't in the best interest of your pancreas, your health, and your weight.

If you woke up with a glucose of 72 mg/dL, and ninety minutes after you ate breakfast your glucose was 90 mg/dL, then whatever you ate was great for your machine. If you woke up with a blood glucose of 100 mg/dL and ninety minutes after you ate breakfast your glucose was 87 mg/dL, then that breakfast was a great fuel choice. I hope this information is making sense to you. Testing provides an opportunity to understand how your body handles what you feed it.

I had an interesting experience recently. I went to Chipotle for lunch and ordered something I never eat: a bowl with brown rice, black beans, grilled veggies (peppers and onions), pico de gallo, lettuce, and a spoonful of guacamole along with an unsweetened iced tea. Most people would think I ordered a healthy lunch because I combined brown rice (a carbohydrate/starch) with beans and veggies. I tested before the meal (glucose 86 mg/dL) and ninety minutes after (glucose 147 mg/dL)! This lunch was clearly not good for me. I was surprised, and yet I wasn't. I knew that combining rice and beans probably wouldn't work for my machine, but I tried it anyway. Beans are considered starchy vegetables; however, they can be a source of protein if you are on a plant-based protein diet. The rice and beans equaled a carb and a protein for my body. I haven't repeated that mistake. If I find myself at a Chipotle, my go-to lunch is a bowl without rice. I have the server add small spoonfuls of either beans or sofritas (tofu), heftier spoonfuls of veggies, and lettuce, topped with guacamole. My machine can handle that.

I think testing is simple and fascinating. Through regular testing ninety minutes after finishing a meal, I have discovered exactly what foods and combinations of food work for me and what work against me. I am practicing self-health. My body is the focus of my research. Listening to my body has provided a wealth of information that has enabled me to keep my body healthy and happy and my weight appropriate. Even if it seems like a hassle at first, testing takes the guesswork out of eating. The more accurate the data, the more effective the lifetime fueling plan.

Adjustment Phenomenon

Please note that some nondiabetic people who have abused their pancreas for many years may in the first two days test within the normal range, 70–100 mg/dL, even though they haven't started DDF. This is because the pancreas is in overdrive due to an unhealthy diet; however, after two to four days of DDF, their blood glucose numbers can register over 100 mg/dL with many fluctuations. This effect can last for several days. Don't worry. It is the body adjusting to a healthier way of eating. Your body will eventually level and represent a realistic picture of what foods it can and cannot handle within a week.

Tuning In

If you are squeamish about pricking yourself or wearing a device like the Libre Pro, then you can *tune in*. Your body is constantly sending you feedback about your health, especially when you eat. Tuning in requires that you get out of your head and truly listen to these cues. Although this method is not as accurate as testing, it will cause you to pause and sort out the feelings you have after eating. Ninety minutes after you eat a meal or a snack, are you tired, starving, and/or irritable, or do you feel energized, wide awake, and ready to enjoy the day? Once you start listening to your body instead of ignoring it, you'll be able to fuel effectively and achieve more positive feelings.

Journaling is just as important for tuning in as for testing— if not more so. In this case, you will journal your feelings upon awaking, after eating, and after exercising/moving. Ninety minutes after finishing a meal or a snack, you will perform a head-to-toe evaluation of your physical feelings and thoughts. If you ate the wrong food (several slices of pizza and a soda), the wrong combination of food (tacos with chicken, pork, steak, or fish along with rice and beans; egg rolls, wonton soup with crispy noodles, and sweet and sour chicken with white rice), or anything that caused your blood glucose to increase significantly (chocolate lava cake with vanilla ice cream), you should feel the ramifications of a pancreas that was forced into overdrive. How will you know?

Remember that insulin and blood glucose do not match up perfectly (if your blood glucose goes up forty points, insulin does not match it forty for forty), and you may experience a major drop in blood glucose (hypoglycemia) due to too much insulin (hyperinsulinemia). These symptoms will help you tune in: *fatigue, rapid heart rate, mood swings, shakiness, headache, dizziness, sweating, nervousness, sleep disruption, hunger (you feel ravenous even though you ate ninety minutes before), difficulty concentrating, and even nausea.* Tune in to your body by setting the alarm on your phone or check your watch ninety minutes after eating. If you feel any of these symptoms, your body is talking to you. It is telling you that what you ate was the incorrect fuel for your organic machine.

If you did not experience any of the above-mentioned symptoms ninety minutes after eating, then more than likely you did not raise your blood glucose levels significantly.

The goal of the DDF lifestyle is to prevent major spikes in blood glucose, thereby avoiding an excessive dump of insulin by your pancreas. Keeping your blood glucose within normal limits will keep your pancreas in "idle mode," not in an overworked state.

Wiser versions of the unhealthy examples above would be cauliflower pizza crust topped with veggies and soy cheese served with a salad and unsweetened iced tea; chicken fajitas with beans or veggie tacos with beans and a salad; stir-fried broccoli and chicken (no rice) or brown rice with tofu and stir-fried vegetables.

It is wise to carry nuts (almonds, walnuts, your choice), a Bobo's Bar (original), a Health Warrior Chia Bar, or some type of healthy snack with you (purse, briefcase, car, backpack) in case you do experience any of the symptoms of low blood glucose. These snacks should bring your blood glucose back within a normal range without significantly spiking it. If you combat the symptoms of low blood glucose with a donut or candy bar, you'll be right back where you started: a significant spike in blood glucose with a huge dump of insulin. It becomes a vicious cycle that causes noncommunicable diseases and weight gain.

Now, if after ninety minutes you *tune in* and feel satisfied, with no symptoms of low blood glucose, then chances are that your blood glucose did not spike and what you ate was the correct meal/fuel for your body. Journaling is critical, as is filling out meal discovery cards so that a pattern of eating appears (see chapter 17 for more information on journaling and meal discovery cards).

Are you are ready to Forget Dieting! and begin a lifestyle of Data-Driven Fueling? If yes, jump in with both feet and don't look back! I'm excited for you and can't wait to hear about your new life.

CHAPTER

6

The Data-Driven
Fueling Program

There are several must-do tasks before you begin the DDF program:

Inform your physician and educate him or her about *Forget Dieting!*

Ask your physician for blood work. A full chemistry panel with fasting blood glucose will provide a baseline. Then have your bloodwork repeated four months later. You and your physician can track the changes, especially if changes need to be made to your prescription medication.

Purchase a scale if you don't have one.

Purchase a tape measure.*

Decide whether you are testing or tuning in.

Purchase the Forget Dieting! Journal or use a notebook.

*Tape measure should be used to measure your upper arms, waist, hips, and thighs before you begin DDF. Remeasure every three months for the first year.

Although I believe in bio-individuality—that we are all different and respond differently to foods—there is a foundation, and the basic tenets of Data-Driven Fueling rest on it.

- Test your blood glucose or tune in to your body cues four to six times per day (depending on how many meals or snacks you have) for three to four months.

- Nothing white—no white potatoes, no white rice, no white pasta, no white flour.

- No refined sugar, artificial sweeteners (Sweet'N Low, Equal, NutraSweet, Sunett, SweetONe, Splenda), or "natural" sweeteners (Stevia and Truvia). Instead, use sweeteners like applesauce, agave, honey, and coconut sugar. Quite often I am asked about Stevia. Stevia is a non-nutritional sweetener derived from a plant found in South America. It has zero calories and is two to four hundred times sweeter than table sugar. So a little goes a long way. Some individuals get stomach issues (diarrhea) from using Stevia. Weight loss has been reported. When I tried it, I was sick to my stomach and had no appetite. My guess is that it's one of the reasons for reported weight loss. Some studies show that Stevia may lower blood glucose. Sounds great, but I'm not sure it is healthy in the long run. It appears that Stevia may have the same effect as Metformin and Glucotrol (glipizide). Both are used to treat type 2 diabetes by causing insulin sensitivity. In laymen's terms, it makes your cells more receptive to the insulin key, which in turn force-feeds glucose to your cells. The glucose leaves your bloodstream, goes into your cells, and lowers your blood glucose numbers. The numbers may look great, but remember, the glucose didn't disappear: it went somewhere. The long-term effects of force-feeding your cells glucose has yet to be researched. In addition, some studies report that alternative sweeteners have been linked to weight gain. Your brain and taste receptors are *partially* satisfied, which causes many to consume more food in order to feel satiated.

Staying away from these sweeteners is the healthier choice. Always remember that less is more. I have told my clients who go to Starbucks and get a caramel macchiato (or similar beverage) and then add sweeteners that if they need all that "stuff" in their coffee, then they don't like coffee. It's time to pick a new beverage.

- No calorie, carbohydrate, or fat counting.

- Avoid dairy (yogurt, cheese, milk, ice cream). *Note:* Children and pregnant women need calcium. Dairy restriction should be determined by patients and their physicians. Calcium-rich foods (kale, for example) and/or supplements may be suggested in place of dairy.

- Limit animal protein (red meat in particular). Many clients are unable to completely swear off dairy or meat, so I tell them to significantly reduce their intake of both. Make Wednesdays and Fridays meatless days. The Physicians Committee for Responsible Medicine states, "Animal protein—in fish, poultry, red meat, eggs, and dairy products—tends to leach calcium from the bones and encourages its passage into the urine. Plant protein—in beans, grains, and vegetables—does not appear to have this effect." Both dairy and animal protein are acidic in your gut and require a buffering agent. The buffering agent of choice is calcium. Because your body is hardwired to survive, it strips calcium from your bones to buffer the steak and cheesy potatoes you just ate for dinner. Due to its inflammatory properties, dairy is especially bad for individuals who have acne, asthma, or cancer.

- Eat fruit separately from other foods, with two exceptions: (1) fruit (apple, banana, pear, or mixed berries) paired with a nut or seed butter, or (2) fruit in a smoothie with protein powder (see recipes in chapter 22).

- Fruit mixed with other foods ferments in your stomach. Mixing alkaline and acidic foods is not good for you. So, the next time you go out for breakfast and the waiter asks whether you want potatoes or fruit with your omelet, say neither or ask for the fruit to go and eat it ninety minutes after you have finished your omelet.

- Practice proper food combining. The basics of food combining are explained in detail in chapter 14.

- Avoid soda, especially diet sodas.

- Drink more water.

- Limit alcohol. Remember, alcoholic beverages like wine, beer, rum, and fruity drinks can raise your blood sugar. If you have a glass of wine, please have a full glass of water before you have a second glass of wine or make a spritzer (mix wine with sparkling water).

- Avoid dried fruits (they have a higher sugar content) and fruit juices.

CHAPTER

7

A Day in the Life of Data-Driven Fueling

"Limitations live only in our minds. But if we
use our imaginations, our possibilities
become limitless."

—JAMIE PAOLINETTI

D o you see where you want to be but have no idea how to get there? I want to help you help yourself. It would be my honor to assist you on your health transformation journey.
A lifestyle change begins with an effective plan that includes a change in behavior (see chapter 9 on behavior modification). That plan requires a schedule in order to facilitate healthy habits. Data-Driven Fueling includes both. Your new schedule will encourage you to eat meals at five-hour intervals with snacks (if needed) in between.

Whether you test or tune in, your meal schedule should look like this:

Begin your morning with a cup of hot water (you can add a slice of lemon). A cup of hot water stimulates digestion and gets your bowels moving.

Breakfast at 8 a.m.., finish at 8:15 a.m., test/tune in at 9:45 a.m.

Snack at 10:30 or 11:00 a.m. (if necessary), test/tune in at noon or 12:30 p.m.

Lunch at 1 p.m., finish at 1:30 p.m., test/tune in at 3 p.m.

Snack at 3:30 or 4:00 p.m. (again, if necessary), test/tune in at 5:00 p.m. or 5:30 p.m.

Dinner at 6 p.m., finish at 6:30 p.m., test/tune in at 8 p.m.

These times are not written in stone. They are intended to give you an idea of what to expect for the next three or four months. After this time, lines of communication between you and your body should be clear. You should have a better understanding of how your body responds to a particular food and not need to test or tune in. You've got your fueling plan.

Also, once you maintain normal glucose levels, your pancreas won't have to work as hard. By maintaining a normal glucose/insulin balance, you will reduce cravings and feelings of hunger.

This is how you should go through your day:

When you wake up in the morning, sit on the side of your bed and take in four cleansing breaths: inhale slowly through the nose, counting 1, 2, 3, 4; hold for a count of four; then exhale through your mouth, counting backward 4, 3, 2, 1.

Go to the bathroom and wash your hands.

Test your blood glucose or tune in and journal the number or your feelings.

Weigh yourself naked (make sure the scale is in the same spot every time you weigh in), and journal it.

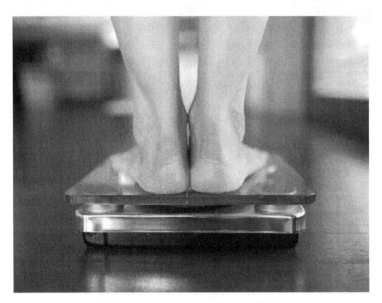

Your body communicates with you all the time.
The number on the scale is one way.

Source: iStock/Getty Images Plus/Phototalk

Pour yourself a cup of hot water. Add a squeeze of fresh lemon juice. This should get your digestive system up and running and stimulate your bowels.

Meditate for ten minutes.

Shower and get dressed.

Then eat breakfast. Remember to set your phone or watch to test or tune in ninety minutes after eating. While eating, please think about how you are going to honor your body and your health for the rest of the day. What will you eat? How will you handle stress? Select foods and beverages that will appropriately fuel your machine, not satisfy cravings. Understanding the basic tenets of Forget Dieting! and food combining makes selections simple. If you know you are having lunch at a particular restaurant, have a plan. Know that you won't be ordering the steak sandwich and fries. Your choice will be a steak salad with dressing on the side and no bread.

Prepare a snack bag of nuts, fruits, or veggies (if you don't snack, you don't have to test or tune in).

Journal what you ate for breakfast and again ninety minutes later with your blood glucose number or tuning-in results.

Take your vitamins.

Eat lunch (selections based on the DDF program/eat to protect your pancreas). Test or tune in ninety minutes after eating.

Do some form of movement/exercise (raking leaves, gardening, walking, yoga).

If you had a stressful day at work or home with the kids, get out and walk, focus on deep breathing, and calm yourself down with soothing affirmations such as "This too shall pass" or "It is what it is." Stress is unavoidable; how we choose to handle it affects our cortisol levels along with our mental and physical health (see chapter 3 on hormones, stress, and weight).

Eat dinner (selections based on the DDF program/eat to protect your pancreas). Test or tune in ninety minutes after eating.

Fill out meal discovery cards and journal before going to bed. Review the day and the day before. Doing so will help you modify your behavior by imprinting activities, food choices, and stress relievers that were positive (should be repeated) and eliminating those that were negative (should be avoided).

Meditate for ten minutes.

Sleep.

CHAPTER

8

Data-Driven
Fueling Calendar

"As I see it, every day you do one of two things: build
health or produce disease in yourself."

—ADELLE DAVIS

Below is a typical Data-Driven Fueling calendar. When you
follow the calendar, you will develop eating habits that
become part of your daily lifestyle. You will reduce and
eventually stabilize your weight and improve your health. You
will consistently provide your body—your living machine—with
the necessary fuel for optimum functioning. The Data-Driven
Fueling calendar takes the guesswork out of daily eating and
allows you to easily follow the Data-Driven Fueling plan.

The Data-Driven Fueling plan does not mean that you can
never have that hot-fudge sundae or piece of cake. Do I drink
wine? You betcha, but I follow a glass of wine with a glass of water
or unsweetened iced tea. Do I eat French fries? Yes, but only once
a month. You are allowed to splurge. "Wild/decadent" meals

should occur no more than two to three times per month (refer to the Data-Driven Fueling calendar).

Remember, your mouth is not supposed to have a party at every meal! You are eating to sustain life, not abuse it! Examples of wild meals would be fried calamari, garlic bread, lasagna, and tiramisu or steak, twice-baked potato, salad with blue cheese dressing, and apple pie à la mode. These wild meals will send your organic machine into a tailspin and screw up your blood sugar, which will lead to a dump of insulin and create cravings that will spin you out of control unless you nip them in the bud.

A wild/decadent meal should always be followed by a liquid fast. The liquid fast after splurging is my take on intermittent fasting. The liquid you decide to drink must have less than five grams of sugar. Either prepare your own or check labels of juices sold at grocery stores. Pressed Juicery has several products that contain less than five grams of sugar.

The liquid fast gives your living machine a break after a wild meal or wild day of unhealthy eating. Taking in only liquids will cleanse and recalibrate your body, preventing you from binge eating and undoing your progress.

The morning after a wild meal will begin with a pressed-greens juice or an apple cider vinegar cleanse drink for breakfast. You will continue to drink liquids as a substitute for meals and snacks. In addition, you should drink water, unsweetened iced tea, or hot tea throughout the day. It is important! You want to make sure you are hydrated properly.

On the following day, return to the Data-Driven Fueling plan for breakfast, lunch, and dinner. For those of you on prescription medication, please speak with your doctor to discuss how your medication might affect your ability to fast. Some medications have hypoglycemia as a side effect, so you don't want to compound that by lowering your blood sugar even more. Remember, never allow your blood sugar to dip below 70 mg/dL.

Schedule: The morning after a wild meal/day, you will begin your liquid fast, drinking something every two hours. Smoothies would be the choice for breakfast, lunch, and dinner. An apple cider vinegar cleanse can serve as your snack drink along with water, iced tea, kombucha, or hot herbal tea. Then the following day you will return to the DDF lifestyle. Recipes for liquid fast days are in chapter 22.

For convenience, I prefer to purchase a one-day juice cleanse from Pressed Juicery. Make sure that you pick low-sugar juices (five grams or less). Evolution Fresh Cold-Pressed Organic Greens & Kale is available in most grocery stores and is low in sugar (four grams). Pressed Juicery's Greens 1.5 has one gram of sugar. Be careful of many other "healthy" smoothies and juices found in the refrigerator section of grocery stores because they contain lots of sugar. Read the nutrition label and check for sugar grams before you purchase. Remember to avoid any that contain more than five grams of sugar.

If you don't splurge on a Friday or Saturday night, you don't have to do the liquid fast the following day.

Meatless Wednesdays and Fridays are self-explanatory: don't eat meat or fish! Choose legumes (beans, lentils, chickpeas, etc.) or soy products (tofu, edamame, etc.) as your protein sources. This gives your digestive tract and your body a break from animal protein. It is also a way for you to reduce global warming.

By eliminating animal protein at least two days per week, you will reduce animal suffering (think factory farming) and global pollution. Animals emit methane and other greenhouse gases in their waste (manure). Animal agriculture is actually responsible for more greenhouse gases than all the world's transportation systems! The United Nations believes gravitating to a more vegan diet is critical to combating climate change.[1]

According to the Environmental Protection Agency (EPA), animals on U.S. factory farms produce about 500 million tons of manure each year. Runoff from factory farms and livestock grazing is one of the leading causes of pollution in our rivers and lakes.

The EPA notes that bacteria and viruses can be carried by the runoff and that groundwater can be contaminated. Many factory farms avoid water pollution limits by spraying liquid manure into the air, creating mists that are carried away by the wind. People who live nearby unknowingly inhale the toxins and pathogens from the sprayed manure.

Commercial fishing such as bottom trawling and long-lining are cited for clearing the ocean floor of life and destroying coral reefs. Fish farms release feces, antibiotics, parasites, and nonnative fish into sensitive marine ecosystems. Keep in mind that most farmed fish are carnivorous. They are fed mass quantities of wild-caught fish. Every pound of farmed salmon produced takes up to three pounds of fish meal feed.[2]

Also keep in mind that 80 percent of all antibiotics are consumed by the livestock industry. This translates into a public health problem because humans are becoming resistant to antibiotics. If your diet consists of mainly animal protein, then you are consuming antibiotics unless you choose antibiotic- and hormone-free animal protein. Therefore, setting aside at least two days a week when you avoid beef, poultry, pork, eggs, and fish will benefit not only your health but also the health of our planet.

SUNDAY	MONDAY	TUESDAY	WEDNESDAY	THURSDAY	FRIDAY	SATURDAY
1 DDF	2 DDF	3 DDF	4 Meatless	5 DDF	6 DDF	7 1 Wild Meal (optional)
8 Liquid Fast	9 DDF	10 DDF	11 Meatless	12 DDF	13 Meatless	14 DDF
15 DDF	16 DDF	17 DDF	18 Meatless	19 DDF	20 DDF	21 1 Wild Meal (optional)
22 Liquid Fast	23 DDF	24 DDF	25 Meatless	26 DDF	27 Meatless	28 DDF
29 DDF	30 DDF	31 DDF				

The Data-Driven Fueling Calendar—your eating plan.

Source: Candice Rosen

Section III

Other Issues
Affecting Health

Behavior Modification

"Your life does not get better by chance,
it gets better by change."

—JIM ROHN

Behavior modification is *the most important factor* in your quest for permanent weight loss and improved health. To properly plug into the lifestyle of Data-Driven Fueling, you are going to have to embrace Forget Dieting! by modifying and changing your behavior. It's the only way.

The term "behavior modification" was first used by Edward Thorndike, an American psychologist, in 1911; however, it was Russian physiologist Ivan Pavlov's principles of classical conditioning that generated behavior therapy, and B. F. Skinner, an American psychologist and behaviorist, ran with it. He formulated the principles of programmed learning and the concept of reinforcement or reward.[1] Behavior modification relies on several principles: *reinforcement* (positive), which serves to increase behaviors, and *punishment* (negative), which serves to decrease behaviors. I don't want you to have to deal with a negative situation such as a heart attack, renal failure, cancer, or obesity in order to change your behavior. I want you to focus on positive behaviors that prevent or reverse a health and/or weight situation.[2]

How you decide to reward positive behaviors will be up to you. A new pair of shoes, a new golf club, a massage, tickets to a concert, or a yoga class may be your reward. Perhaps knowing you were able to reduce your consumption of animal protein by 50 percent last week or the fact that your physician lowered your dosage of blood pressure medication or insulin will be enough compensation. The ultimate reward is to *Forget Dieting!* because you understand how to care for and feed your organic machine.

People are often skeptical. They have attempted to make changes in the past. Trying out new diets, joining health clubs, plugging into rigorous workout routines, engaging in significant food restrictions with the expectation of permanent results only to be disillusioned when they eventually end up where they started—who wouldn't be skeptical?

Serial dieting is beyond frustrating. It's so much easier to give up or not even try. Most diets don't work because people who engage in a particular diet have no clue how food truly affects their health and weight. Dieters don't incorporate the new "diet" into their lives because it's a temporary solution. Few think of diets as a lifestyle. They lack an understanding of how their body processes what they eat and how it affects their weight and health. They have failed to replace old habits with new permanent habits.

How is the *Forget Dieting!* approach to weight loss and improved health better than other programs? It eliminates the cycle of "yo-yo" dieting. Strong psychological and motivational attitudes about weight can exacerbate this cycle for many. Frustration over not achieving either the desired amount of weight loss or the desired body shape can contribute to a negative attitude before you even begin a new program.

These experiences, along with mobility issues, often color an individual's contemplation of trying yet another diet. For individuals with obesity who suffer from osteoarthritis, cardiovascular disease, or chronic back or joint pain, physical limitations can contribute to a vicious cycle of depression and further weight gain due to inactivity. I want you to know that even with a physical disability it is still possible to lose weight and reverse noncommunicable diseases (NCDs) on the DDF program. Many of my clients have mobility issues, and yet they still lose weight and improve their health. The key is to change your thought processes and your behaviors around food, and your mobility issues will improve. Remember, you are fueling at every meal, not dieting!

If you want to change your weight and your health, then you have to change your attitude. It's the truth, and your life depends on it. You have to put food where it belongs as a necessity to operate your body/organic machine. The fuel your body burns twenty-eight out of thirty days of the month should be "clean" fuel. It's not easy considering all the temptation out there, and it isn't easy to think about caring for yourself when you are so busy; however, you have to make yourself and your health a top priority.

It's only human nature to want a shortcut. In this day and age, we are beyond overwhelmed due to work and family responsibilities. There are not enough hours in the day, and we usually end up last on our list. Therefore, any shortcut is welcomed. Unfortunately for too many, their physical appearance and health issues reflect that lack of self-care and failure to practice self-health.

So who has time to focus on eating healthily and working out? Fast food, diet pills, prescription medication for health issues, delivered prepared meals, bariatric surgery, and quick solutions promised by fitness and health experts all power the search for someone or something to make life easier. Never forget that quick fixes are Band-Aids that mask issues and symptoms; they do not address root causes or provide lasting solutions.

Although we gravitate toward easy and quick solutions, studies of people who have achieved permanent weight loss indicate that a particular diet is only a small part of success. Of greater importance are the adoption of long-term goals, personal determination and discipline, and a restructuring of eating and exercise habits.

Most people hate change. Right? It takes effort, and there is a fear of the unknown. Even if your situation is bad, you've developed a certain comfort level over the years. The devil you know is better than the devil you don't. Life is ever changing, and since we have limited control over that, many people I've worked with feel a sense of comfort in sticking with eating habits that are unhealthy. They know that Kentucky Fried Chicken, a Starbucks caramel macchiato, or a Big Mac from McDonald's is always going to taste the same, and that is comforting. These familiar foods will contribute to health and weight issues, but there's comfort in the taste. So why change?

Your behavior-modification goal is to instill more appropriate and positive behaviors and to recognize triggers that sabotage good choices. If driving past McDonald's makes you want to stop and order a Big Mac and fries, take another route. If you know that ice cream is a self-soother for you, then make sure you don't have any in your freezer. Or find a different way to soothe yourself—a cup of flavored tea, a ten-minute meditation, a walk outside. The goal is to replace a bad habit with a good one, and then reinforce the good habit by repeating it.

Basically, diets make daily food decisions for the dieter who, upon returning to his or her old eating habits, nearly always regains the lost weight. Some of the quick weight-loss programs produce mostly a loss of body water, not fat. In fact, the initial rapid loss during the first week or two is primarily fluids as the body adjusts to utilizing its stored fat. Then the dieter stops losing as quickly as he or she did on first starting, becomes frustrated, and quits.

Diets are usually geared toward a short-term goal rather than a long-term one. Australian researcher Samantha McEvedy stated that people expect to get something out of dieting, despite knowing it usually won't work.[3] I understand the skepticism; however, those wanting to improve their health or lose weight have to understand that they are both the problem and the solution.

Behavior modification is tricky. If you are like me, you want to make changes; yet it is extremely hard to turn off old habits, taste buds, cravings, and daily routines that are influenced by food and pharmaceutical companies. These saboteurs have brainwashed us and woven their way into our lives via television commercials and strategically placed ads. We are creatures of habit and mass marketing.

Marketing is now geared toward the idea that heavy is sexy and overweight is the norm. Morbidly obese teens are told to celebrate their fullness, to embrace the beautiful you, the big you, and to be proud. Those promoting this view fail to explain the future health issues these teens will be forced to deal with as they age.

Many schools contribute to this decline in health by eliminating daily gym and recess. The childhood obesity epidemic is partly their fault. All of it adds up to a distorted view of what is normal, a decline in the value of health, billions spent on unhealthy food, and an overburdened health-care system.

Parents need to understand that they are responsible, more than ever before, for the weight, health, and well-being of their children. Childhood obesity and type 2 diabetes are at epidemic levels in the United States. Type 2 diabetes mellitus has long been considered a disease of adults and is associated with increased risk of cardiovascular morbidity (unhealthiness) and mortality (death).

During the past ten years, an increasing frequency in the occurrence of type 2 diabetes mellitus has been reported in children (eight-, nine-, and ten-year-olds) and adolescents. I discussed this subject before, but I can't stress it enough. This increase of type 2 diabetes parallels the increase and severity of obesity in children and adolescents.[4] Children who are obese are at a significantly elevated risk for adverse health outcomes, including both physical and psychological problems. The most common medical comorbidities associated with obesity include metabolic risk factors for type 2 diabetes, such as high blood pressure, high cholesterol, impaired glucose tolerance, and metabolic syndrome. Orthopedic problems, sleep apnea, asthma, dental problems, and fatty liver disease are also common in obese children and adolescents.[5]

Setting achievable weight-loss goals has several important benefits for individuals and families with obesity. If you have children, perhaps the stimulus for you to change will stem from your concern for them. You don't want your children to suffer from preventable diseases. Your decision to no longer participate in the insanity of eating your way to poor health and obesity will benefit everyone around you, especially your children.

Even when you have the best intentions, certain situations and problems can interfere with your behavior-modification plans. Interpersonal relationship issues, job-related troubles, health issues, and financial struggles can impact your daily life and attitude. This is only compounded by the constant bombardment of negative news about communities, cities, states, countries, and the world.

Letting go of what you cannot control is the first step in the right direction. The next step is acknowledging what you do have control over: *what you put in your mouth, how much you move,* and *how you deal with stress.* Celebrate those decision-making privileges and make them count.

Socioeconomic factors play into behavior modification too. My father was a steelworker, and my mother was a homemaker. There were no credit cards back then. Because my parents lived from paycheck to paycheck, dining out was a rarity. And when we did dine out, we had McDonald's, Kentucky Fried Chicken, or pizza. This was inexpensive compared to dining at a restaurant, and it was a break for my mom and a "treat" for us.

Equating fast-food meals with possible health issues was not on my parents' radar. Too many families in this country eat this way because it's cheap and easy. Cheap is actually expensive. You end up paying for that meal in poor health, weight gain, medical care, and prescription medications. The presumption that you have to be wealthy to eat well is a falsehood. We ate healthier when my mom purchased a chicken, roasted it, and served it with a salad.

The cost in 2019 of a typical "don't have time to cook" fast-food dinner of burgers, fries, and drinks for four is approximately $28. If you stop at the grocery store on your way home from work and pick up a precooked chicken ($8–$9), a bag of prewashed salad ($4), and some broccoli ($5), your cost will be approximately $18 (assuming you have oil and vinegar at home for salad dressing). You definitely don't have to be rich to eat well. False marketing interferes with behavior modification.

Many clients have expressed acceptance of their weight and health. Those with that mind-set blame genetic factors ("my mom and dad are overweight") or traditional ethnic eating ("I'm Italian, and this is the way we eat"; "I'm Mexican, and I can't give up beans and rice").

You may have to modify multigenerational ethnic recipes, along with your thinking about what constitutes a healthy meal. No more lasagna with garlic bread or burritos with meat, beans, and rice. Family obesity is a significant issue in the United States. Family food history is important and can compound the problem. How did your family shop for, cook, and eat food?

My grandparents came from villages in Europe. Their eating habits were completely different. Meat was a luxury. Smoked meat was used to flavor beans and cabbage, for example. Lunch would consist of a salad and two boiled eggs. My parents' generation had access to grocery stores (unheard of in the "old country"), and processed foods (after World War II) changed the way my mom shopped and how we ate.

My grandmother (who lived with us after my grandfather died) developed health issues (diabetes and heart disease) that her parents in the old country never experienced. My dear mother suffered from the same. A massive heart attack at age sixty required a quintuple bypass, which led to hospitalizations for congestive heart failure. The offshoot diseases of type 2 diabetes continued with diabetic retinopathy, renal failure, and circulatory issues in her legs. Plans were made to amputate a leg prior to her death at age seventy. My mother suffered for ten years, but she wasn't the only one. All of us who loved her suffered as well. It took a toll on the whole family.

Approximately fourteen years ago, I changed my family health history. I stopped shopping, cooking, or eating like my grandmother (after she came to the United States) or my mother. My mother died nineteen years ago, and after her death I was responsible for my dad until he died (2018) at the ripe old age of ninety-six. Several years ago, he complained, "You know, you don't cook like your mother." I replied, "That's right, old man, and that is precisely why you are still alive." I have put food in its proper place as a source of fuel. My food choices reflect clean fuel, not junk. I modified my behavior to reflect my new mind-set. I don't ever want to compromise my health or that of my family with poor choices. Parents and families need to understand that their familial origins and cultural histories have an impact on their food preparation. Healthier versions are in order to help themselves and their loved ones.

I'd like to address a subculture of people I've come across who actually like going to the doctor. They like the attention; their health issues and medications are a topic of conversation with family and friends and many times provide an excuse for avoiding certain situations. These individuals have to work particularly hard at changing their behavior because the positive reinforcement (sympathy, attention, or the use of health as an excuse to avoid something) is of immediate value to them. If this is you, I think it's important to work with a therapist. Exploring the root causes of that mind-set is important. I think talking about how you transformed your health and your weight is so much more interesting than discussing health problems. Trust me, no one really cares or wants to hear about your aches, pains, medications, physical therapy, or what your doctor told you.

I suggest that some of my clients think of themselves as addicts. Food is their drug of choice. As they avoid their food addictions, they may experience withdrawal. This is especially true of sugar. The withdrawal is both physical and emotional. And just like any addict, they can overdose. Obesity and NCDs are obvious neon signs of overdosing. Remember, your weight, health, and quality of life depend on kicking your food addiction and embracing a new mind-set around eating.

Do you have faith in yourself and your ability to change? Do you believe your body is willing and waiting to partner up with you? If you've gotten to this chapter, I think you are ready to Forget Dieting!

Let's start with modifying your conception of food. I'd like you to write down what meaning food has for you. How were meals handled in your home? Did everyone sit down together for dinner? Were meals eaten on the run? Did your mom cook? Is food your go-to soother when depressed or angry? Assessing long-held thoughts about food and eating is critical. How does food play out in your life? As you improve your health and reduce your weight, go back and reread what you initially wrote and reflect on your past and present thoughts about food. Are you still eating, or are you fueling? Write about that transformation.

As I stated before, I believe in the practice of self-health. You have to commit to being your own healer. You have to believe that your weight, health, and well-being are first and foremost your responsibility. I believe the essence of behavior modification is practice. You have to practice proper fueling. The more you practice making correct fueling choices, the more ingrained they will become in your lifestyle. Practicing Data-Driven Fueling on a daily basis will alter your mind-set about what your body needs to operate. This will lead to healthier habits.

Dr. Loretta Graziano Breuning states in her book *Habits of a Happy Brain*, "Old habits are like well-paved highways in your brain. New behaviors are hard to activate because they're just narrow trails in your jungle of neurons. Unknown trails feel dangerous and exhausting, so we're tempted to stick to our familiar highways instead."[6] Be bold—venture onto a new trail! As the saying goes, the journey starts with a single step.

Be Objective about that Reflection

You have to be objective about what you see in the mirror. Really do a total assessment of yourself. Take off all your clothes and stand in front of a full-length mirror. What do you see? This is not about shaming; it is about communicating with your body. Would you say you are in fairly good shape? Could you lose a few pounds, or have you morphed into someone you no longer recognize? Seeing oneself through totally distorted "glasses" and adapting to the new norm (big is beautiful; "I was born this way") is something that each and every one of us has to fight against. It's a form of apathy. If you have been struggling with weight issues for years, that prevents you from seeing who you really are. If you've suffered from high blood pressure, high cholesterol, or type 2 diabetes for many years and been on various prescription medications, you probably don't remember how it feels to be healthy and off medication. You can't recall a life without an umbilical cord connected to your local pharmacy.

Outline Your Goals

What are your goals? What do you want to change or improve upon? Do you want to lose thirty pounds? Do you want to walk a mile? Do you want to get off prescription drugs or significantly reduce the dosage? Do you want to sleep better? Do you want to feel better? Do you want to wear your belt around your waist instead of below your belly? Define five goals and then write down what you believe you need to do to achieve them. Remember, it is not just about the weight. It is about health. Behavior modification will work in your favor.

Many individuals living with obesity and health issues experience self-blame, low self-esteem, and general negativity about themselves and their situation. It's not your fault. How can you help yourself if you don't know how to? With so many diet programs out there, how could anyone possibly figure out which one is best? Forget Dieting! takes the mystery out of the care and feeding of your body. You just need to make a commitment to fueling and follow the program.

I encourage baby steps, not giant leaps, as you transform yourself. Changing your eating habits along with your mind-set about food, nutrition, celebrations, and movement/exercise is a lot to take on. I don't want you to set yourself up for failure. Baby steps are less uncomfortable and less disruptive, especially if the whole family is planning to Forget Dieting!

For some of you, "dieting" has created unhappy memories. Those memories affect your ability to modify your behavior. Maybe you have tried many diets, exercised extensively, and only lost a small amount of weight, or maybe you reached your goal and then, the moment you strayed from the diet or reduced your exercise time, found yourself back in the same position you started at. A change in eating or movement that doesn't incorporate behavior modification will never last. Remember, Rome wasn't built in a day. Slow and steady wins the race. Adopting this approach to achieve weight loss and improved health will work in your favor rather than "I need to lose ten pounds in a week." Slow and steady, accompanied by imprinted behavior changes, will lead to sustainable healthy habits.

A change in behavior that results in positive results reinforces the sustainability of weight loss and the reversal of NCDs. Increased self-confidence as you see improvement should convince you that the mentality of "dieting" instead of Data-Driven Fueling is a dead end.

Here are some DDF behavior-modification tips I want you to incorporate into your life:

1. Practice self-love for your body, mind, and spirit.
2. Eat to sustain life, not destroy it.
3. Be mindful—before you eat anything, ask yourself, "Will this abuse my pancreas and organic machine?" If the answer is yes, don't eat it.
4. Less is more—do you really need the huge steak, baked potato, or burger and fries? Or would a simple salad with sliced avocado and kidney beans or thin slices of steak on top be a better DDF option?
5. I can do anything I set my mind to.
6. My mind has to think of my body and my spirit when making decisions.
7. Taste with your mind and your memory. Most people know what a hot-fudge sundae or apple pie à la mode tastes like. Savor those memories and protect your health by not eating it.
8. Ignore television commercials for fast and processed foods. The goal of these companies is to make money and rob you of your health. They know what they're selling isn't healthy. It is up to you not to be a victim.
9. If you have to take a deep breath before your next bite, you know you are finished with that meal! Always leave something on your plate. Don't clean the plate.
10. Eat slowly—don't rush through a meal; savor it.
11. Avoid using food as a reward.
12. Use the *rubber band technique*:

    Place a rubber band around your wrist. Every time you find yourself in a situation (pondering a tuna melt versus a salad, looking at a dessert menu, placing a gallon of ice cream in your grocery cart—any unhealthy choice), I want you to snap that rubber band against your skin. You need to get your attention. When you've been snapped back to DDF reality, I want you to replace whatever negative choice you were about to make with a positive one that reflects your DDF lifestyle.

    The rubber band is a form of behavior modification. It serves to get your attention in order for you to consciously choose a new behavior that will eventually become your new healthier habit. Snap away until the DDF lifestyle is woven into your thoughts, actions, behaviors, and beliefs.

The Data-Driven Fueling Calendar will aid in behavior modification by helping you build new eating pathways. It's repetition. You know how you will eat each day of the week. If it's Wednesday or Friday, you know those are vegetarian or vegan days. After several months, your brain and behavior can't help but modify your choices and create healthier habits. You've built a new highway in your mind about eating. It isn't a dirt path. It is a road poured with precision nutrition concrete.

1. Set weekly goals (e.g., one to two pounds of weight loss per week). What steps will you take? You might walk fifteen minutes an hour after dinner, eat less animal protein, or try a new healthy recipe.
2. At the end of the week, review your journal. Did you meet your goals? If yes, what helped you succeed? If no, what affected your ability to achieve your goals? What can you do next week to improve on the previous week? Remember to reward yourself (but not with food!).
3. What behavioral changes have you made?
4. Put Post-it notes on your refrigerator and bathroom mirror to remind yourself of your commitment: "Your mouth is not supposed to have a party at every meal!" "Think before you eat!" "I love me." "I eat to protect my pancreas." "I don't diet, I fuel."
5. Identify triggers and replace them with healthier options and soothers: "I feel sad" (call a friend); "I'm craving sweets" (cut up an apple and spread crunchy almond butter on it); "I'm angry" (move—jump rope, take a walk); "I'm bored" (go to the movies, get off the couch, or clean out a closet).

The focus of behavior modification is to decrease negative behavior, increase desired positive behavior, and in the end create a healthier lifestyle. An example: "I plan to increase my activity this week. I plan to walk two miles on Monday, Wednesday, and Friday." How will you do this? In the morning, afternoon, or evening? Will you do it by yourself or with a friend? Make sure you have the proper shoes and clothing and take a water bottle. Make sure you eliminate barriers that will stop you before you begin.

The most effective techniques for behavior modification are goal setting (set realistic goals: one to two pounds of weight loss per week); self-monitoring (through glucose readings or tuning in to feelings and physical activity journaling); contingency planning (keep small packets of raw almonds handy and sprinkle them on a salad if dinner is at a pizza place); stimulus control (I had a fight with my girlfriend, and I want nachos and a beer); positive reinforcement (I didn't sit on the couch last night and eat potato chips, so I'm going to get a pedicure); cognitive restructuring (a healthy dinner is NOT a steak, salad, and baked potato); problem solving (I'm going on a cruise, and the buffets are so tempting, so what is my plan?).

Don't forget to reward yourself for making positive changes. What will your reward be at the end of a week? What new goals will you set? If you were unable to achieve your goals, what happened? What could you have done differently?

The major behavior reinforcers are the reversal of NCDs and weight loss. We each have the ability to live life with courage, compassion, and good health. Inner transformations enable us to push ourselves to be our best. This inner transformation is much like a personal revolution. You are revolting against what has brought about weight gain and poor health. You are revolting against misinformation and long-held beliefs. It will be a daily battle until it becomes your new norm. There is no going back because the foundation of DDF is your new foundation. These changes are now interwoven into what you eat, how much you move, and how you deal with stress. The more open you are to change, the easier it will be. Trust me.

"You are always one decision away
from a totally different life."

—UNKNOWN

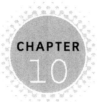

Movement

> "Life is like riding a bicycle—in order to
> keep your balance, you must keep moving."
>
> —ALBERT EINSTEIN

D o you like to exercise? Are you active daily or five out of seven days per week? If not, you should be. I like to refer to exercise as "movement" because every time clients hear the word "exercise," they cringe and become defensive about why they are unable to do it.

I believe so many people don't engage in exercise and avoid it at all costs because they consider it a chore or punishment. They procrastinate with a million reasons as to why tomorrow is better than today to plug into movement.

I am a baby boomer, and at age sixty-five, I am unable to do many of the exercise routines proposed by millennials and contemporary fitness gurus, but that's okay! Instead of running or signing up for a kickboxing crunch super bootcamp, I found movement that works for me: yoga, swimming, hiking, horseback riding, tennis, gardening, golf, and housework.

Typical exercise programs require one to carve out a specific time and place for a workout. Many people are unable to adhere to a schedule because "life happens." And that's completely valid! So let's shelve the 4:45 p.m. aerobics on Wednesday and focus on daily movement. Adding movement into the daily routine you already have is easy and accomplishes what you want to do: burn up fuel before it gets stored.

Think of your body as your house and your joints as its furniture or its nooks and crannies. What happens if you don't dust your furniture or clean around the baseboards or corners of a room? You get an accumulation of dust, dirt, and cobwebs, right? Think of your hips, knees, shoulders, and other joints as items you need to "dust." Moving prevents the formation of "cobwebs" in your joints. Moving keeps you flexible. The goal is to avoid ending up like the Tin Man from *The Wizard of Oz*.

I put music on while I cook, and then I dance. I do deep knee bends every time I take clothes out of the dryer. One article of clothing at a time, so if there are ten pairs of socks in the dryer, that equals twenty deep knee bends. I know where the items are at my local grocery store (where I park in a faraway spot to get a little extra walking in); however, I purposely create my shopping list in a manner that requires me to go from one end of the store to the other for each item. Every step adds up. Every single time your body moves, it burns glucose (the body's fuel). When you eat correctly to protect your pancreas and move, your body must go into your storage tanks for extra fuel, which leads to weight loss.

As long as you engage your body in some physical activity, you are ahead of the game. Remember, the added benefit of movement/exercise is the release of endorphins that aid in reducing stress, anxiety, and depression and increase sleep, self-esteem, and flexibility.

Choose movement/exercise activities based upon what you enjoy. You will repeat rather than avoid a pleasurable activity. I love hiking in the mountains near our home. I'm not in a race. Hiking up a hill is strenuous, and I accomplish more in a shorter distance than on a long horizontal walk. I make it a point to listen for different birdsong and take notice of trees and flowers. When I visit my two youngest children in New York City, I can walk over twelve thousand steps without realizing it because I am so absorbed by the buildings (the different architecture), people, and storefronts. If I set out to walk x number of steps, it would become a chore, and I would be disappointed if I did not reach my goal. That's how my mind works. I just set out to hike or walk and enjoy the process.

Whether it's a New Year's resolution or a summer tune-up, each and every one of us starts out with good intentions. However, when we make goals that are unrealistic, overly complicated, or overwhelming, we end up stressed and discouraged when we don't achieve them. This can lead us to self-sabotage. We eat the wrong foods to alleviate stress and instead raise our stress hormone levels by worrying about the activity we hate participating in and our unwise dietary choices.

The wrong movement/exercise can become counterproductive for some. What do I mean by that? Some of my clients experience a significant rise in their blood glucose when exercising because stress is associated with the activity. If you are in a yoga class and you stress over your inability to do a pose properly, you can trigger your body into that fight-or-flight response and negatively impact what you are trying to achieve: weight loss and improved health. If you don't like riding a bike, do not participate in a spin class just because your friend is doing it. Otherwise your stress will impede your progress. If an activity is too difficult for you and makes you unhappy, don't do it.

I am also a nonbeliever in vigorous/strenuous exercise—especially if you have more than forty pounds to lose. The DDF reasoning behind that is this: if you work on building up muscle before losing the weight you need to lose, adipose (fat) tissue becomes compressed between your muscles and skin, which I believe makes losing weight harder. After losing the desired amount of weight, you can increase your exercise/movement and add weights or resistance bands to better define your muscles and sculpt your body.

I recommend establishing a simple movement routine that feels manageable to you. Even just ten to fifteen minutes per day of movement can reduce your weight and improve your health;

you can even break up longer amounts of movement into shorter bursts throughout the day. Find a movement/exercise/activity that you enjoy so that you create a healthy addiction. Healthy habits become healthy addictions when you do them every day. I want you to become addicted to health! Your healthy addictions begin with Data-Driven Fueling, followed by exercise/movement and stress reduction.

When making decisions for your body, make sure your thoughts revolve around what will help it operate at an optimal level. You know that how much exercise you do doesn't matter if you continue to eat an unhealthy diet or have poor eating habits; you're just treading water. You know that an unsweetened iced tea is better for you than a sweetened one. You know that movement is better for your organic machine—your muscles, bones, ligaments, heart, and lungs—than sitting on a couch. Intrinsically, you know the answer. Make each day count.

The following are simple exercises/movements you can do without a gym membership or between trips to the gym:

1. *Hula hooping.* I have lower-back issues, but since I started yoga and do appropriate exercises to strengthen my back and abdominal muscles, I can hula hoop. Buy a weighted hula hoop. If you don't remember how to hula hoop or never attempted hula hooping, search for a demonstration on YouTube. Put on your favorite song and go for it! I like to hula hoop to "Ride like the Wind!"

2. *Walking.* Yes, I know you hear it all the time. But walk! I enjoy an early-morning walk because it sets me on the right health course for the rest of the day. It puts me in touch with my body and creates a desire to nourish my machine properly throughout the day. You can also walk before or after dinner. If you walk after dinner, wait forty-five to sixty minutes after eating to allow your body to digest your meal before you walk. Being outside is also good for your mental health and mood.

3. *Doing squats.* In order to perform proper squats, remember to have the heels of your feet "glued" to the floor to prevent

unnecessary pressure on your knees. As you get into a squat, make sure your back is straight/flat and your chest is up. Remember that it is OK to steady yourself by holding on to the top of the dryer or a stable object nearby. Aligning your back and chest prevents your knees from receiving too much pressure and reduces the strain on your lower back. Your core also benefits from this simple movement.

4. *Swimming laps or jogging in shallow water.*
5. *Biking* (in your neighborhood or on a stationary bike).
6. *Dancing.*
7. *Exercising to a DVD at home.* I love Richard Simmons's *Sweatin' to the Oldies.* Maya Fiennes's Kundalini Yoga DVD focuses on strengthening the adrenal glands and kidneys (very important components in stress reduction). My daughter turned me on to Callan Pinckney's Callanetics DVD.
8. *Doing yoga/Pilates.* If you don't want to join a yoga studio, you can access some very good yoga programs on YouTube.
9. *Playing tennis.*
10. *Jumping rope.*
11. *Jumping jacks.* Yes, start with ten or twenty and work up to fifty or one hundred.
12. *Doing yard- or housework.* Vigorous housework can equal a trip to the gym. Scrubbing the floor for forty-five minutes or an hour burns up four hundred calories.
13. *Boxing.*
14. *Weight lifting.* I use eight-pound weights and do arm repetitions (twenty to thirty bicep curls for each arm and twenty to thirty tricep kickbacks—You Tube provides tutorials).
15. *Hiking or bowling.* An incredibly motivated mom in our community established a Friday hiking group. She picks out the hike and e-mails us all. It is stress free. We all hike at our own pace. The ages of the hikers range from twenty-nine to seventy (I'm the second oldest!). In addition, my friend Michele and I organized a bowling league. We are not serious bowlers, and neither are the other twenty women, but we have so much fun, and we move!

Whether you get down on your hands and knees to wash the floor, hula hoop, wash the windows, wash your car, lift weights, dance, or walk after dinner, any of the activities will raise your heart rate, increase stamina, and force you to utilize muscles that need to be dusted off and engaged.

Create a checklist or refer to the Forget Dieting! Journal. Before you go to bed, make sure that you have accomplished your goals for the day. Those should include protecting your pancreas, listening to your body, moving, reducing stress, and Data-Driven Fueling.

I cannot emphasize enough the need to love and care for yourself. Put yourself in your top five. Remember, your mind, body, and soul are in a partnership, working in unison to make your time on this planet pleasant. By engaging in some activity on a daily basis, you add to the positive.

You have the inner knowledge; you know what to do. It's actually harder not to do it because that ten- to fifteen-minute walk will be spent elsewhere, like waiting in line at your local pharmacy for medication for a disease whose cause is rooted in poor food choices and inactivity. It's up to you. But I have faith in you. I know you can change. I know you can move, and I know your new DDF lifestyle will inspire others. You will become a beacon of light.

The Importance
of Sleep

A good night's sleep is essential to the overall well-being of your organic, living machine. This means at least seven to eight hours of sleep at night for adults and more for children and adolescents. Just as if you left your car running nonstop without providing proper maintenance, lack of sleep will cause your body to deteriorate. The body requires the restoration you can only obtain through sleep. Your heart, lungs, stomach, intestines, kidneys, nerves, and especially your brain need a break. Every cell in your body needs some downtime.

Humans spend about a third of their lives sleeping. Scientists believe that the most important reason for a good night's sleep is memory consolidation. In today's world, our brains are overwhelmed with information and stimulation. How does the brain retain everything it is exposed to in a given day? Well, researchers theorize that sleep allows the brain to sort through information and selectively choose what it needs to store.

There are five stages of sleep. The first is drowsiness, when your eyelids become heavy; your head starts to drop, and you feel sleepy. It is a time when you can be easily woken up because your brain is still active, tuned in. This period lasts about one to seven minutes.

The second phase is light sleep, when your brain activity begins to slow down and your eyes stop moving; however, you are not in a true sleep and can still be easily woken up. This phase lasts approximately ten to twenty-five minutes.

The third and fourth phases are intertwined, each lasting between twenty and forty minutes. The body is sliding toward a deeper sleep, a time of non-rapid eye movement (or NREM). During this phase it wouldn't be easy to wake you up.

The fifth stage, called the REM (rapid eye movement) cycle, may be familiar to you. During REM sleep, the brain begins to wake up. It is the phase when dreams happen. Your eyes may be rapidly moving, but the muscles of your body are "paralyzed." Sleep research shows that during this stage many individuals experience between three and five dreams a night.

Each of our bodies has an internal clock, a cadence referred to as the circadian rhythm. It is a biological clock set by sunlight's blue light. Although people often associate blue light with computers, fluorescent lights, compact fluorescent light bulbs, phones, and LED lights, the largest source of blue light is the sun. Blue light affects the body's circadian rhythm, our natural sleep and wake cycle.

Blue light stimulates us and wakes us up by hitting special receptors in our eyes, which trigger the pineal gland, often referred to as the "third eye." This small gland located deep in the center of the brain is shaped like a pine cone and secretes melatonin, which plays a role in the body's internal clock.

Melatonin secretion is highest during dark nighttime hours and lowest during daylight hours. This is why many people who have trouble sleeping take melatonin supplements. So you can imagine why light exposure can wreak havoc on your sleep. It is important to ensure that your bedroom is dark.

Many electronic devices produce enough light to reset your biological clock, but using backlit screens late at night can confuse your brain, preventing the production of melatonin and delaying your sleep. That is why it is important to leave your electronic devices (cell phones, iPads, etc.) in another room.

Insufficient or restless sleep may suggest an underlying health problem such as gastroesophageal reflux disease (the backup of stomach contents into the esophagus) or sleep apnea (abnormal breathing pauses). Lack of sleep can place you at risk for heart disease, diabetes, obesity, and depression. It is important to speak with your physician to rule out health problems.

The *European Heart Journal* reported that a lack of restful sleep can increase the risk of developing or dying from heart disease by 49 percent and stroke by 15 percent.[1] There is evidence of a connection between sleep, stress, and metabolism. Sleep deprivation, chronic exposure to stress, and overeating lead to the increased incidence and prevalence of metabolic disorders such as obesity and type 2 diabetes.[2]

A poor night's sleep can also affect your cognitive abilities. There is a strong relationship between dementia and lack of sleep. A study published in the medical journal *Neurology* stated that individuals have increased risk if they get less sleep during the REM phase. Researcher Dr. Matthew Pase and his team found that people who took a longer time to reach the REM sleep stage and who spent less time in the REM cycle were at a greater risk of developing dementia.[3] In addition, Taiwanese researchers Drs. Hung Chao-Ming and Li Ying-Chun and their team found that patients with primary insomnia, especially those under forty, had a higher risk of developing dementia than those without primary insomnia. Sleeplessness causes deficits in brain function. It's a fact.

What adds to sleeplessness is prescription medication for noncommunicable diseases. Certain medications are sleep influencers and can affect sleep negatively.

- *Alpha-blockers:* used to treat high blood pressure, benign prostatic hyperplasia, and Raynaud's disease (a rare disorder affecting blood vessels, usually in the fingers and toes, which respond to cold or to stress by narrowing, which limits blood flow to the surface of the skin).

- *Beta-blockers:* prescribed for high blood pressure, abnormal heart rhythms, angina, migraines, tremors, and certain kinds of glaucoma.
- *Corticosteroids:* used to treat inflammation of blood vessels and muscles, rheumatoid arthritis, lupus, Sjögren's syndrome (immune system disorder identified by its most common symptoms—dry eyes and a dry mouth), gout, and allergic reactions.
- *Selective serotonin reuptake inhibitor (SSRI) antidepressants:* SSRIs treat symptoms of moderate to severe depression.
- *Angiotensin-converting enzyme (ACE) inhibitors:* used to treat high blood pressure and congestive heart failure.
- *Angiotensin II–receptor blockers (ARBs):* used to treat coronary artery disease or heart failure in patients who are unable to tolerate ACE inhibitors or have type 2 diabetes or kidney disease from diabetes.
- *Cholinesterase inhibitors:* used to treat memory loss and mental changes in patients with Alzheimer's and other types of dementia.
- *Nonsedating H1 antagonists:* commonly known as antihistamines (they stop the body's production of histamine) and used for allergic reactions (itching, sneezing, runny nose, watery eyes, nasal congestion, and hives). This type of H1 antagonist does not cause drowsiness like first-generation antihistamines (Benadryl).
- *Glucosamine/chondroitin:* used to improve joint function, relieve joint pain, and reduce inflammation.
- *Statins:* used to treat high cholesterol.

That is why it is so important to address the root causes of health issues. Otherwise you can experience a domino effect. If an unhealthy diet has caused high cholesterol and the need for a statin drug, which in turn is affecting your sleep and may result in dementia, doesn't it makes sense to change what you eat? Rather than causing a *negative* domino effect, you can bring about a *positive* domino effect just by modifying what you put in your mouth.

A National Institutes of Health–funded study found that prescription sleeping pills reduce the average time it takes for an individual to fall asleep by approximately thirteen minutes, compared to individuals given a placebo. Interestingly, participants in a sleep study believed they had slept longer than they really had, by up to one hour; however, the sleep time was only increased by eleven minutes.[4] This is thought to be due to anterograde amnesia, which causes trouble in the formation of memories. When people wake up after taking sleeping pills, they may simply have forgotten they were unable to sleep. If sleeping pills only increase total sleep time by about eleven minutes, are they really worth it when you consider the side effects?

Furthermore, medication only masks sleeping issues. Treating the root cause is much more effective in the long run. Are you stressed or worried by a particular issue or situation? Did you drink too much alcohol? Did you drink caffeine before bed? Did you have to get up to use the toilet because you drank too much? Are your prescription medications making it hard for you to sleep? It is important to think about what might be contributing to your insomnia.

A National Sleep Foundation survey discovered that 43 percent of people between the ages of thirteen and sixty-four reported lying awake at night due to stress.[5] It's hard to think clearly when you haven't rested properly! Today's stressors include work, the death of a loved one, divorce, loss of a job, financial problems or obligations, getting married, moving, illness or injury, emotional problems (depression, anxiety, anger, grief, guilt, low self-esteem), taking care of an elderly or sick family member, and traumatic events (natural disaster, theft, rape, violence).

Stress can also come from within. Are you a worrier? Do you fear things you have no control over—terrorist attacks, toxic chemicals, global warming, war, politics, and the future? Unrealistic expectations or a negative attitude toward or perception of events or actions (even happy ones) can cause stress. Perhaps you are someone who doesn't deal well with change. Whatever the issue, the result is worry, and it leads to stress, which creates an unhealthy state for your sleep and your body.

Stress causes a reaction in the body; remember the fight-or-flight response? The body responds via the autonomic nervous system with a heightened state of arousal for extended periods. This state of alertness due to stress can generate anxious thoughts, thereby delaying, disrupting, or reducing sleep. The lack of restful sleep only adds to the stress factor. This vicious cycle can also affect your appetite. Sleeplessness can arouse hunger.

In late July 2016, the Global Council on Brain Health hosted a meeting in Toronto, Canada, to translate the scientific evidence on sleep and brain health into actionable recommendations for the public.[6]

They suggested that lack of sleep may cause the following:

- Premature aging
- Slowed reaction time/decreased coordination (think car accidents)
- Decreased ability to learn
- Depression
- Memory issues
- Increased mood swings
- Increased risk of Alzheimer's disease and dementia
- Decreased immune system function
- Increased stress and an inability to cope with it
- Decreased athletic ability
- Decreased ability to think clearly

The brain of a sleep-deprived individual is similar to the brain of an individual in deep sleep. Why? Because the brain is *less active.*

The following are a few things you can do to improve your sleep:

- Avoid daytime naps (especially for older people). If you must, only nap for twenty to thirty minutes and not in the evening! A longer nap or a nap too late in the day will affect nighttime sleep.

- Avoid prescription sleeping pills, as they can have major side effects, including disorientation, confusion, amnesia, and hallucinations. They can also increase your risk for insulin resistance, weight gain, diabetes, and food cravings.
- Prepare your sleeping nest (your bedroom and your bed) to be conducive to sleep. Do you have a comfortable mattress? A comfortable pillow? How about your blanket? Do you need a body pillow? Does your significant other snore?
- Be sure your room is dark.
- Pick a bedtime. Have a sleep routine that you stick to every night, with exceptions only for special occasions. Going to bed and waking up at the same time provides a routine that the body craves. I know that if I go to bed after 11:30 p.m., I will not sleep well.
- Try taking a hot bath before bed. Hot baths have also been known to lower blood sugar levels. Dr. Steve Faulkner of Loughborough University found that a soak in the tub reduced peak blood sugar levels by 10 percent more than an hour of cycling.
- Switch off the television.
- When you get into bed, bring your thoughts into a state of gratitude: you have a roof over your head, you are safe, you are warm, you are cozy—yes, in so many ways, you are lucky.
- Some people swear by sound machines; let the sound of waves or a thunderstorm lull you to sleep.
- Turn off all blue screens one hour before your planned bedtime.
- Use a weighted blanket. According to the National Sleep Foundation, weighted blankets can help people with insomnia and anxiety. The extra weight can feel like a hug. Warning: *Never* use a weighted blanket on a baby or toddler!
- Get a "kiddie blanket." Many department stores (e.g., T.J. Maxx, Marshalls) carry extremely soft little blankets in the infant section. I tell my clients to buy one and place it on top of their pillow. The softness is very comforting and soothing.

- Meditate for ten minutes before bed. Meditation apps are available as well as YouTube.
- Avoid arguments before bed.
- Turn down the thermostat. It is better to be in a cool room rather than a warm room.
- Some researchers say to keep pets (dogs and/or cats) out of the bedroom and definitely off the bed. I disagree. For many, having their pet(s) in bed provides a level of comfort. Our dog Pearl shares our bed.
- Avoid caffeine and alcohol for at least two to three hours before bedtime. Alcohol may cause you to "pass out," but you will not have a restful sleep.
- Take a fifteen-minute walk at least forty-five minutes to an hour after dinner and at least an hour before bed.
- Some researchers believe that sleeping in the nude improves the quality of sleep. There are no binding garments, and the body temperature is cooler without pajamas.
- Leave your phone in another room—unless you are using it to listen to a meditation or guided imagery app.
- No laptops in your room. Leave your computer in another room.
- Dot your pillow with lavender oil.
- Read something light before going to bed. Stress-provoking material will not promote sleep.

Melatonin and Valerian

Melatonin and valerian root are supplements used as sleeping aids for sleeplessness and jet lag. They are not a cure for insomnia. You will have to experiment with both and see which one works best for you.

Melatonin

In 2001, the Massachusetts Institute of Technology found that 0.3 mg of melatonin is sufficient to restore peaceful sleep in adults.[7]

However, the National Sleep Foundation recommends a dosage of between 0.2 mg and 5 mg for adults each day. Still another school of thought is if you are over twenty years of age, the suggested dosage is 3 mg. If you are over forty years of age, the dosage can be increased up to 5 mg. Again, speak with your physician before taking any over-the-counter medications or supplements.

Valerian

A study conducted found patients taking valerian had an 80 percent greater chance of reporting improved sleep compared with patients who took a placebo. Valerian root may interact with alcohol, some antihistamines, muscle relaxants, psychotropic drugs, and narcotics. If you are taking any of these, please use valerian only under the supervision of a physician. Valerian may increase the sedative effects of anesthesia and should be discontinued at least one week before a surgical procedure. Again, speak with your physician.

The recommended adult dosage of valerian is one teaspoon of tincture in a quarter cup of water or one to two capsules (between 400 mg and 1,000 mg) at bedtime. Discuss the dosage with your physician.

Moon Milk

Although some health-care professionals do not advise liquids before bedtime due to the disruption of sleep with a trip to the bathroom, ayurvedic medicine believes warm milk is a remedy for sleeplessness. I personally enjoy an occasional cup of Moon Milk[8] before bed when I have trouble sleeping. Here is the recipe for one serving:

1 cup unsweetened almond or hemp milk

½ teaspoon ground cinnamon

½ teaspoon ground turmeric

¼ teaspoon ground ashwagandha (or another adaptogen, like shatavari or astragalus)

2 pinches of ground cardamom

1 pinch of ground ginger

1 pinch of ground nutmeg

Freshly ground black pepper (to taste)

1 teaspoon virgin coconut oil

Honey (no more than ½ teaspoon) *(optional)*

Bring milk to a simmer in a small saucepan over medium-low heat. Whisk in cinnamon, turmeric, ashwagandha, cardamom, ginger, and nutmeg; season to taste with pepper. Whisk vigorously to incorporate any clumps. Add coconut oil, reduce heat to low, and continue to cook until warmed through, about five to ten minutes (the longer you warm it, the stronger the medicine). Remove from heat and cool slightly. Stir in honey to taste (avoid cooking the honey, or you'll destroy its antibacterial healing properties). Pour into a mug and drink warm, and then go straight to bed!

A good night's sleep is critical to weight loss and the health and well-being of the brain and the body. The maintenance of your organic machine is dependent on adequate sleep. Addressing and exploring the root causes of insomnia will only add to the long-term benefits of the Data-Driven Fueling lifestyle.

Sabotage

"Our ultimate freedom is the right and
power to decide how anybody or anything
outside ourselves will affect us."

—STEPHEN COVEY

M*acmillan's Dictionary* defines the verb "to sabotage" as
"to deliberately stop someone from achieving something
or to deliberately prevent a plan or process from being
successful."

Sabotage is a serious issue for some embarking on the journey toward weight loss and improved health. Friends, coworkers,
and, yes, even loved ones can be threatened by the emerging new
you. A friend who has given up on losing weight due to yo-yo
dieting may not be supportive of your decision to Forget Dieting!
and change your lifestyle. Your spouse may view your new look
as a threat to the marriage, thinking, "He/she might leave me for
someone else." Or, perhaps more innocently, maybe your spouse
liked it better when you ate bad foods together and sat on the
couch for movie night.

Your dieting changes may make others feel that your new lifestyle is adversely affecting their lives. You're a killjoy because you don't want to go out after work for pizza and beer. You may be excluded, without malice, from social events because you are now making conscious decisions about what you put in your mouth, and it makes friends feel bad about their choices. Or worse yet, they may tempt you with "Just a little won't hurt."

I have warned many a client about sabotage. They didn't believe me until they experienced it themselves. Yes, several clients' loved ones actually sabotaged their attempts to lose weight and improve their health. Sounds crazy, right?

I'd like to share stories about two clients. One woman I worked with began to experience issues with her husband. She had lost forty-five pounds and felt great; her physician had eliminated one of her medications and significantly reduced the dosage of the other. She was so excited at one visit because she had purchased a pair of jeans in a size fourteen. She was thrilled because she hadn't worn jeans in years. Well, her husband was so "proud" of her weight loss and improved health that he felt she deserved a "treat" for all her hard work. So he brought home a hot-fudge sundae for her. She thanked him but refused to eat it. The ensuing months brought about food temptations and accusations of infidelity. When she was fat and on medication, he had nothing to worry about. Her metamorphosis threatened him on every level. His insecurities and jealousy overshadowed any pride he felt in her accomplishment. Whether deliberately or subconsciously, he worked hard to undermine her efforts. The result was the same: he sabotaged her.

Client number two was a sixty-six-year-old male with insulin-dependent type 2 diabetes. He came to see me because he wanted to lose weight, reduce his intake of insulin, and prevent any further damage to his eyes (due to diabetic retinopathy). He also wanted to be more active. He couldn't walk a block. After four months of eating to protect his pancreas, his insulin intake was significantly reduced by two-thirds; he lost weight, had more energy, slept better, and was able to walk one mile from the train to his office. He looked fantastic and was in great spirits. His wife felt "sorry" for him and the "sacrifices" he was making, so she rewarded him by stocking the kitchen with all his favorite foods—the same foods that got him into his previous state of health. He was also a victim of sabotage, even if his wife's actions were "well intended."

An important question to ask yourself as you embark on your Forget Dieting! lifestyle is: How supportive will family members, friends, and coworkers be when you announce your lifestyle change? Will they be respectful of your decision? Will they avoid tempting you? And if tempted, will you be able to deal with the saboteurs?

I can tell you from experience that family, friends, and coworkers will want to know how your change will affect them. As with an alcoholic who decides to stop drinking, friends and loved ones will want to know how the *new* you will affect their fun and their lives.

I myself have had many people over the years make comments like "I think you're too thin," "There's no fun in eating like you," "I put a cheese platter out, but I know Candice will disapprove," or "I shouldn't order this because Candice is here." I laugh it off. Anyone who knows me knows that I never make anyone feel uncomfortable, whether I'm a guest in their home or we are out for dinner at a restaurant. It's their life. The life I have chosen is one free of doctor's appointments and prescription medicine. Healthy fueling is a small price to pay.

Most people don't like change. When you are no longer the friend who goes out for burgers, cheese fries, and beers after bowling, that can upset the friendship applecart.

I counsel my clients to be prepared for sabotage. Family members, friends, and coworkers, especially if they are in poor health or overweight themselves, are *not* going to like your announcement and the resulting transformation, or they just plain won't get it. It is up to you to educate everyone who has a place in your life and in your heart about your lifestyle change. They may be clueless that offering you a piece of pie is a form of sabotage (they mean well). They may have no idea that rewards for improving your health and losing weight are completely unnecessary. Food should never be a reward for practicing self-health. So you must excuse them; don't stress over it. However, if once informed of your new way of fueling your organic machine these well-meaning souls continue to tempt you, then you must be firm that *you* have made a lifestyle choice and you would appreciate their support.

This lifestyle choice is not a diet plan to lose *x* number of pounds. This is the way you intend to fuel your body based upon solid data for the rest of your life. Your body has spoken about what it wants to be fed. It is not your intention to judge their way of living; you just decided to make a healthy change. You are fueling your body with what it needs, not feeding it what it wants based on stress, a taste you have, food corporations' marketing, or your friends' and family's expectations.

If a friend, family member, or coworker offers you a tempting treat, just reply, "Thank you, I really appreciate that, but I'll pass this time." Or you can say, "Thank you, but I'm full and couldn't eat another bite." If they continue to push something on you, take it, tell them you'll save it for later, and then pitch it in a garbage can when they aren't looking.

I cannot stress it enough: Your body is not a dumpsite. It is an organic, living machine, and it requires the correct fuel to run at optimum efficiency. Anyone who doesn't care about your weight, health, or well-being should be put on notice or avoided. When I say "put on notice," I mean you have to be very clear that you are honoring yourself and won't comment on their choices; therefore they need not comment on yours. You would appreciate their support and would be more than happy to share with them what you have learned. Above all, do not give in when someone offers you a "treat" or feels bad for you because of your sacrifice.

That funny friend is still in you, just without the extra weight. As you change your weight and your health, you may no longer be the friend who doesn't pose a threat to go out with. Yes, I've known women in the past who like to go out with their overweight friends rather than their in-shape friends to increase their chances of getting hit on. Sad but true.

What about self-sabotage? Some of you know what I mean. Think about celebrities, musicians, and athletes who, once they reach what they have been striving for their whole lives, end up doing something to completely undermine everything they ever worked for. Perhaps the praise, respect, success, adulation—whatever noun you want to use—doesn't feel right and becomes an uncomfortable, ill-fitting outfit to wear.

Success, whether professionally or personally, can feel uncomfortable. Get over it and get comfortable as you transform your body and your health. Your DDF lifestyle is all about the caring and feeding of your organic machine.

If you have worked hard to become more active, lose weight, and wean yourself off medication, why would you turn on yourself? The cruel "anti-self" undermines our desires, casts doubts on our abilities, and convinces us to be paranoid and suspicious of ourselves and others, says Dr. Robert Firestone in *The Enemy Within*.

Why would anyone want to go back to square one and return to a practice they don't want? Self-sabotage happens all the time. The question of why we act against ourselves is a difficult one to answer.

Early life experiences form our critical inner voice. Whether your critical self-sabotaging came from parents, grandparents, teachers, or peers during your childhood or teenage years, it is time to replace that critical voice with a supportive one.

What to do? You have to be connected to what *you* want. I know you have worked hard in the past to lose weight and improve your health; yet you find yourself back where you started because of "yo-yo" dieting. It's frustrating and depressing—I get it—but you have to engage your mind to work in unison with your spirit and your body. If your dream is to be healthier and/or to lose weight, then defeatist thinking isn't going to help you convince your body and your spirit to join you in your quest to make your dream a reality.

If your goal is to lose twenty-five pounds, but your thoughts veer toward negativity ("that's an impossibility, I've tried dieting before"; "I've been heavy my whole life, Forget Dieting! isn't going to work for me"; "high blood pressure is in my DNA"), then your thoughts will sabotage your goals.

If you state that your goal is to get off high blood pressure medication, then your thoughts must focus on what you need to do to make that happen. Changing the way you eat is one action; moving/exercising is another. Your thoughts also need to include your desire to Forget Dieting! You have to believe that what you knew before was about dieting and what you know now is about fueling. It's a lifestyle, and you are not going to let anything or anyone (including yourself) undermine your future health.

The mind has to reboot and become the cheerleader of the body and the spirit. Author Elizabeth Gilbert said, "You need to learn how to select your thoughts just the same way you select your clothes every day."[1] Before you go to bed at night, write something nice about yourself or a nice thing you did that day and write down your plan for the next day.

If your mind takes off down a negative path, I want you to think about what your body and spirit might say about that. If your mind has made a decision to eat a slice of deep-dish pizza, consider what your body and spirit might think about that choice.

Every decision you make has to take into consideration the other two components and your ultimate concept of how you want to live and feel. Before you decide not to move/exercise or before you decide to stuff that cupcake in your mouth, I want you to pause and consider the other two "voters" in the decision-making process. If the mind is the only one voting yes, then the choice is a definite no!

You have to love yourself and engage your entire being to work in unison to make your dreams happen. What will you select from your arsenal of behavior-modification tools? Have you decided that because it's Wednesday, you'll refrain from eating any animal protein? Will you walk an extra fifteen minutes? If donuts are on the coffee station table at work, what are you going to do to avoid the temptation? Will you embrace a positive attitude if you do deviate from the Data-Driven Fueling plan at lunch or fall down a rabbit hole? As changes in thinking occur, please compliment yourself on the courage, strength, and determination you are incorporating into your life.

As you commit to the Forget Dieting! lifestyle, self-sabotage loses power. The critical voice is slowly silenced because you have no choice when it comes to your health. It is your duty to care for and fuel your machine properly. Ignoring the signals and abusing your machine is no longer an option.

Tips to Reduce Sabotage

- Your mind, body, and spirit work in unison and are interdependent.
- The proper care and fueling of your machine is an essential part of your daily routine.
- Your new lifestyle is about fueling, not eating!
- Anyone interfering with your lifestyle will be politely informed that while their support is valued, any temptations are unwelcome.
- There's no going back; Forget Dieting! You've been there, done that—not anymore.

Tips for Dealing with Saboteurs

- Reassure them that your lifestyle change is for you. You are not trying to convert anyone (although I'm hoping that you will). Your feelings for them haven't changed.
- Reiterate that your lifestyle change is to improve your health first.
- Suggest they join you in some of your new activities.
- Politely or jokingly decline repeated efforts to get you to have that drink or that donut. "No thanks" should be enough, but if they keep going, find your "pat" answer or change the subject.
- Stick with your decisions firmly. Change is not easy and can cause insecurity in those you hold dear, even if they are supportive on the surface.

- Bring a healthy item to a gathering. Example: bringing a fruit or veggie platter to a brunch when you know others are bringing donuts and croissants.
- Drink sparkling water with a lime from a wine glass at a party or restaurant—it's festive and may reduce the anxiety others feel that you're not joining in on the drinking.

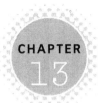

CHAPTER

13

Addictions Other Than Food: Drugs and Alcohol

When my son read this chapter, he said, "Mom, why are you writing about this? Does it really belong in your book?" I think it does belong in *Forget Dieting!* Over the years I have had clients who overconsume alcohol or indulge in regular or recreational drug use and wonder why they can't lose weight. Both drugs and alcohol affect weight, health, and sleep.

People take drugs to feel better (to reduce anxiety, physical pain, and depression), to feel good (more self-confident, energetic, or relaxed), to do better (to enhance sport performance or improve concentration in school or at work), or out of social pressure or curiosity.[1]

Anytime alcohol or drugs are used as props in order to cope with underlying issues, you have a problem. Addressing the root cause of the problem is the first step. Do you hate your job? Are you in a stressful relationship? Is your self-esteem low? Do you suffer from anxiety? Are you depressed?

Drugs are both a personal health issue and a public health problem. The opioid crisis is a case in point. Senseless deaths due to drug overdoses or excess alcohol (think high school and college kids who die from alcohol poisoning, car accidents, choking on their own vomit, or a fall) affect not just loved ones left behind but also public health. When the mind is altered and clear thinking is absent, we are all at risk.

Illicit drug sales instigate inner-city violence. More violent crimes have happened because people were under the influence and not of sound mind. Many of the homeless in the United States are addicted to drugs and/or alcohol. Typhus is currently a public health issue with the homeless population in downtown Los Angeles. Drug use induces a sense of apathy and altered state of reality (cleanliness is not always a top priority), which is a threat to the individual's well-being and the community at large.

Research has shown that people who drink alcohol consume it three to four times a week; yet those who use marijuana use it seven days a week. That's seven days too many to be under the influence.

Eleven states and the District of Columbia have legalized marijuana for recreational use, and thirty-three states have legalized it for medical use. This development has been met with great joy by many; however, marijuana is not a benign substance. The American College of Obstetrics and Gynecology had this to say in 2017: "Because of concerns regarding impaired neurodevelopment, as well as maternal and fetal exposure to the adverse effects of smoking, women who are pregnant or contemplating pregnancy should be encouraged to discontinue marijuana use." Yes, babies can be born with neurological issues, premature, and even stillborn if you smoke marijuana. Those who use it for nausea just might have to deal with that sensation rather than cause irreversible damage to the child they are carrying.[2]

Again, marijuana is not benign. It is notorious for creating the munchies. Marijuana will make you fat! In fact, it significantly increased total daily caloric intake by 40 percent![3]

Your appetite is increased, and that puts your health and weight-loss goals on the back burner. I'm amazed when I hear individuals lecture about the state of our planet, global warming, and pollution, and yet, as they speak, they are polluting their own bodies with drugs, inappropriate food, and alcohol.

Although studies that showcase the benefits of wine (in particular red wine) have merit, the researchers did not have their study subjects down a bottle by themselves. So why do people overdo it with alcohol? Well, people drink alcohol for a variety of reasons:

1. It is accessible; it's even sold at grocery stores.
2. Lots of family members and friends drink.
3. It's an act of rebellion (for underage drinkers, defying the rules is a rite of passage).
4. There's an element of peer pressure (as your friends are all ordering cocktails before dinner and having a bottle or two of wine during dinner, you go along with it).
5. It's fun (it makes some people more animated, "the life of the party").
6. A party is often thought to be more fun if alcohol is served and everyone's drinking.
7. It can reduce feelings of stress (albeit only temporarily).
8. Past experiences have been positive (if you were the "life of the party" and it felt good, you'll resort to alcohol at the next social event).
9. It's socially normal (if alcohol consumption in your community is woven into the fabric of events—weddings, Fourth of July, book club—then you plug into that without thinking).
10. Marketing pushes it (movies, television commercials, and shows connect liquor with urban chic).
11. Any sporting event is a beer-drinking opportunity (tailgating).

Scientists have discovered that alcohol switches the brain into starvation mode, increasing hunger and appetite. In fact, modern studies confirm that alcohol intake acutely stimulates eating and correlates with obesity. So if you binge drink, expect to binge eat![4]

Drugs and the overconsumption of alcohol may provide temporary relief from a whole slew of issues, but they have a negative impact on your organic machine by raising your blood glucose, heart rate, and blood pressure. They can cause sleep issues, accidents, inappropriate behavior, liver damage, and inflammation of the pancreas; they can also affect a fetus (pregnant moms beware) and even cause various cancers. In any case, it is estimated that one in every four deaths is caused by drugs and alcohol, according to the World Health Organization. My guess is that the true number is actually higher, with some deaths being attributed to other causes (injuries sustained in a car accident).

It is more important to be clearheaded and able to think rationally. Nothing in life is ever solved by drug or alcohol use. Life is difficult. Unfortunately, sad, challenging moments may outweigh happy ones, but life should never be defined by an expectation of perfection. Life is not "a bed of roses." Anyone can deal with perfection. That's easy. It's actually when the shit hits the fan, when you face adversity, stress, and unhappiness, that you find out what you are made of. Tackling difficult situations and issues with solid coping skills reduces the likelihood of resorting to a substance crutch.

I'm not saying not to drink, although I am saying that you should avoid drugs. I enjoy my wine; however, I don't overwork my pancreas, compromise my health, and alter my thinking with excess. Keep in mind when drinking alcohol that both excessive daily drinking and binge drinking are unhealthy. Rule of thumb: up to one drink per day for women and up to two drinks per day for men. If you choose to have a glass of wine over dinner, please remember to follow the glass of wine with a full glass of water or unsweetened iced tea.

I believe you know that poisoning your body with food, alcohol, and/or drugs is unhealthy and your body deserves better. So don't allow your mind to make choices that negatively affect your body and your soul. There is help out there: local substance abuse centers, Alcoholics Anonymous, your primary physician, clergy, friends, family, self-help books—you just have to reach out.

Remember, the only true power you have is what you put in your mouth. Appreciate this option of choice, and use it to respect and honor your body. It is your best friend and willing partner. Recognize that relationship as you pursue your Forget Dieting! lifestyle.

Section IV

Data-Driven
Fueling Toolbox

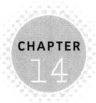

CHAPTER

14

Basic Food Combining

F ood combining, also known as "trophology," is a nutritional approach that recommends specific combinations of foods. Born in 1877, Edgar Cayce was known for his contributions to the connection between diet and health, particularly with regard to food combining, the acid/alkaline diet, and the therapeutic use of food. Dr. Herbert M. Shelton's 1951 book *Food Combining Made Easy* and William Howard Hay's 1920 book *The Hay Diet* showcased the benefits of proper food combinations.[1]

Food combining is a simple approach to eating based on the way your body digests specific foods. Every macronutrient (fats, carbohydrates, and proteins) digests at a different speed. These macronutrients require the release of different digestive solutions and enzymes to break down what you have eaten. Opposing foods combined in the same meal have conflicting digestive requirements, which is considered bad for you and your gut.

Let's take pasta with meat Bolognese, for example. Protein (the meat in the sauce) requires an acidic environment to digest (utilizing the digestive enzyme pepsin), while carbohydrates (the pasta) require an alkaline environment (utilizing the digestive enzyme ptyalin). Since pasta and meat have opposing digestive requirements, combining them in the same meal will cause the

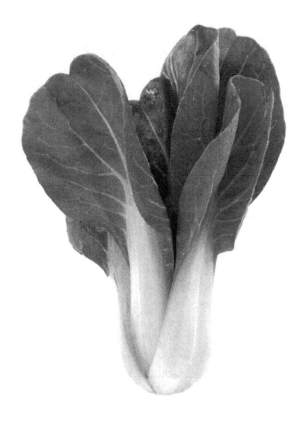

Source: © iStock/Getty Images Plus/lujing

body to release both acid and alkaline enzymes. Acid and alkaline solutions neutralize each other, which slows down digestion.

When you improperly combine foods, you confuse the body. The body throws out several digestive enzymes to deal with the various food choices. This will slow down digestion and deplete the body of digestive energy, causing feelings of sluggishness, bloating, and gas.

When individuals complain of "gut issues," perhaps the issue isn't a lack of probiotics but improper food combining. Think about it: If your digestion is slowed down due to an improper combination of foods, your body will have to deal with a chemical imbalance. This chemical imbalance leads to prolonged digestion, which can cause food to putrefy and ferment in the stomach and intestines. This is an unhealthy situation for your organic machine because undigested food particles can end up in your bloodstream and may even cause food sensitivities.

Non-starchy vegetables and leafy greens have their own digestive enzymes and digest much faster than starches, proteins, and fats, which means they can be paired with any food combination without causing a toxic environment in your gut. Because they are not high in natural sugars like fruit (especially dried fruit: raisins, apricots, etc.), they don't cause gastric disturbances.

Elementary Food Combining

Proper food combining makes breakfast, lunch, and dinner choices simple.

When creating a meal, choose a main component from one of the following categories. That choice will be the *primary* base of your meal. You will choose a protein (animal or plant-based), a starch, or a fruit as your **base** from the following lists:

Proteins
Animal Proteins

Fish	Poultry
Red meat	Eggs
Pork	

Plant-Based Proteins
Tempeh
Tofu
Beans (black, kidney, cannellini, lentils, chickpeas)
Meat substitutes (Tofurky, Gardein, Boca, MorningStar, etc.)

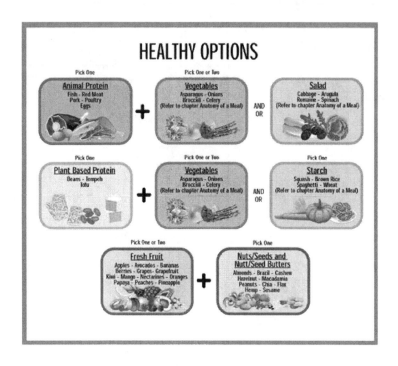

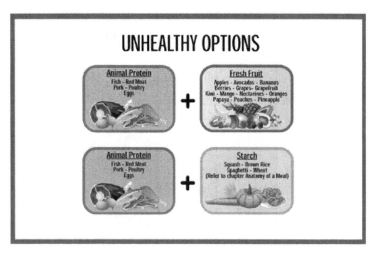

Starches

Acorn squash
Barley
Butternut squash
Brown rice
Brown rice pasta
Buckwheat
Farro
Lentils
Millet
Oats
Quinoa
Rye
Spaghetti squash
Spelt
Sprouted grain bread or English muffin (may include barley, spelt, or millet bread)
Sweet potato
Wheat berries

Fruits

Apples
Avocados*
Bananas
Berries
Grapes
Grapefruits
Kiwis
Mangos
Nectarines
Oranges
Papayas
Peaches
Pineapples
Pomegranates

*Avocados are nutrient dense and may be used as a base (half an avocado with almond slices for a snack) or a garnish (omelet with a couple of slices of avocado). Avocados are also a healthy fat.

After picking just *one* selection from one of the above groups, you can add items from the remaining groups of vegetables, nuts, and seeds to round out your meal.

Vegetables

Artichokes
Asparagus
Alfalfa sprouts
Arugula
Bamboo shoots
Beets (sparingly)
Bean sprouts
Beans (green, wax,
    yellow)
Bok choy
Broccoli
Broccoli rabe
Brussels sprouts
Butternut squash
Cabbage
Cauliflower
Celery
Chicory
Cucumber
Chinese cabbage
Collard greens
Corn (uncooked)
Carrots (sparingly
    and uncooked)

Dandelion greens
Eggplant
Endive
Escarole
Fennel
Garlic
Ginger
Green cabbage
Red cabbage
Jicama
Hearts of palm
Kale
Jalapenos
Kohlrabi
Herbs (parsley,
    cilantro, basil,
    rosemary,
    thyme, etc.)
Iceberg lettuce
Leeks
Mushrooms
Okra
Mushrooms
Mustard

Onions
Peppers (green,
    red, yellow,
    orange)
Radishes
Romaine
Radicchio
Scallions
Shishito peppers
Spinach
Shallots
Swiss chard
Sugar snap peas
Snow peas
Tomatillo
Tomatoes
Turnips
Yellow summer
    squash
Sauerkraut
Water chestnuts
Watercress
Zucchini

Nuts

Almonds
Brazil nuts
Cashews

Hazelnuts
Macadamias
Peanuts

Pecans
Pistachios
Walnuts

Seeds

Chia	Hemp	Sesame
Flax	Pumpkin	Sunflower

For a more extensive list of fruits, vegetables, and nuts for proper food combining, visit my website: www.candicerosenrn.com.

Undefined Exceptions

Why is it important to (usually) eat fruit alone? Fruit is fast digesting, and when it is eaten along with protein or starch, the digestion is hindered. The fruit can ferment in your gut, which can cause indigestion, bloating, and gas. Eating fruit alone ninety minutes before or after a meal is the healthiest way to incorporate it into Data-Driven Fueling. So when you order that egg-white omelet and the waiter asks whether you would like hash browns or fruit, by all means ask for the fruit; just wait ninety minutes to eat it.

However, as I stated before, you can combine nut butters, nuts, seed butters, or seeds with a fruit. You can add fruit to a smoothie as long as you include a healthy fat (plant-based protein powder, nut/seed butter, or avocado). You may try serving fruit on a bed of plain spinach, arugula, or romaine with a sprinkle of nuts or seeds—see how your body responds.

Remember, if you choose fruit as a meal or a snack, you cannot combine it with dairy (yogurt or cheese), protein, or starch no matter what. You must eat it alone, with a nut or seed butter, or with a quarter cup of nuts.

I have included beans and lentils in both protein and starch categories. I use beans as a protein source (vegetarian chili is an example). Because beans are a vegan protein, I serve them with a baked sweet potato (a carbohydrate). This combination does not raise my blood glucose. Sweet potatoes are low in carbohydrates and have a low glycemic index rating.

Even though many people think eggplant is a vegetable, it is actually a fruit. In my eating plan, I use it as a vegetarian option for entrees. I love eggplant sauce over brown rice pasta or zucchini pasta.

Avocados can be combined with a starch and with a protein. Their fat content appears to slow the glucose spike. A snack for me would be 10–15 tortilla chips with guacamole. I would use avocado in a quinoa salad, sliced on top of an omelet or mashed and spread on sprouted-grain toast.

You can use butter, ghee, grape seed oil, and olive oil. Healthy fats include avocados, eggs (organic, free-range), seeds (pumpkin, sunflower, sesame, chia seeds), nuts (walnuts, almonds, cashews, pecans, peanuts), extra virgin olive oil, and coconut oil. Non-dairy items include nut and soy cheeses (cheddar, mozzarella, cream cheese, etc.); unsweetened almond, cashew, coconut, rice, or soy milk can be used as you wish.

Remember these rules: leafy greens and non-starchy vegetables go with everything!

Main meals should be eaten at five-hour intervals (remember the chapter on digestion):

Breakfast—8:00 a.m.
Lunch—1:00 p.m.
Dinner—6:00 p.m.

Data-Driven Fueling is truly a no-brainer. Your organic machine will let you know what fuel works best for your body. Listen observe and incorporate the information into your decision-making!

CHAPTER

15

The Anatomy
of a Meal

"Viewing this meal as medicine, I shall enjoy
it without greed or anger, not out of gluttony
or out of pride, not to fatten myself
but only to nourish my body."

—TIBETAN BUDDHIST PRAYER
OFTEN RECITED BEFORE A MEAL

E very meal should reflect an understanding of what your
body and, most important, your pancreas can handle. The
key to constructing a meal is to understand the basic foundation of Data-Driven Fueling and to master food combining.
Once you have processed what constitutes a healthy meal that will
benefit rather than impair your organic machine, you can dine in
or out without having to worry about your health or your weight.

In pursuit of the DDF lifestyle, the anatomy of a meal is your
personal research study of the internal workings of your body and
how it processes what you have chosen to eat.

Constructing a healthy meal is simple. I will show you how easy it is to make the correct choices and to say no to incorrect ones. It's about avoiding the following:

- Anything white (white flour bread, white flour pasta, white potatoes, white rice, white sugar)
- Dairy (cheese, yogurt, milk, ice cream)
- Sweets (donuts, cakes, cookies)
- Sugars (artificial and regular)
- Sodas (diet or regular)
- Cooked corn
- Fruit eaten with other foods
- Any foods you see advertised on television
- Processed foods
- Stress/emotional eating
- Improper food combining

And it's also about combing food according to Data-Driven Fueling: never eat an animal protein with a starch. Examples include roast leg of lamb with potatoes; chicken and rice; eggs with hash brown potatoes; pasta with meat Bolognese.

A foundational principal of Data-Driven Fueling is that fruit is always eaten alone/separately with a few exceptions: fruits can be combined with nuts or seeds or nut/seed butters, and they can be used in a nondairy smoothie. Examples include the following: a smoothie with Vega protein powder, kale, unsweetened almond milk, blueberries, and strawberries; a bowl of berries with a heaping tablespoon of almond butter.

Examples of good food combinations:

Protein:

Wild salmon + broccoli + mixed green salad

Organic ground turkey Bolognese + zucchini "pasta" + mixed green salad

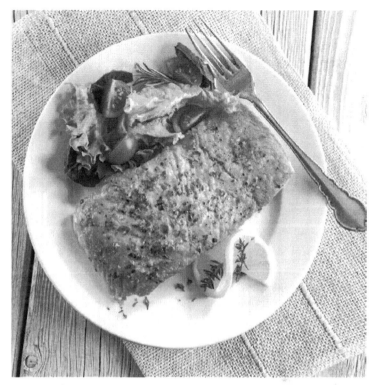

An example of proper food combining (the lemon is a garnish).

Source: © E+/alle12

Grilled or baked chicken + sautéed kale or mashed cauli-flower + mixed green salad

Starch:

Quinoa + avocado + hearts of palm on a bed of arugula

Butternut squash soup (made with vegetable broth) + charred brussels sprouts + mixed salad

Brown rice pasta + eggplant marinara sauce + mixed green salad

Baked sweet potato + black beans + arugula salad

A bad choice would be chicken parmigiana with linguine and marinara sauce (animal protein + carb/white flour pasta + mozzarella). Another bad choice is pancakes or waffles with bacon or sausage (carb + animal protein).

Main meals should be eaten at five-hour intervals:

Breakfast—8:00 a.m.

Snack—10:30–11:00 a.m.

Lunch—1:00 p.m.

Snack—3:30–4:00 p.m.

Dinner—6:00 p.m.

These times are approximations. If you need to have snacks between meals, then you would have your first snack at 10:30 a.m. or 11:00 a.m. and the second at 3:30 p.m. or 4:00 p.m.

Nuts and seeds may be used as complements to salads and fruits. A few examples: half an avocado served with slivered almonds on top, an apple with cashew butter, sprouted-grain bread with almond butter.

A word about dried fruits (raisins, cran-raisins, apricots, dates, figs, prunes, etc.): Avoid them or eat/use them sparingly because the sugar content is too high. The same goes for fruit juices.

As you commit to the DDF lifestyle, you will find blurry areas. Even though avocados are referred to as fruits, the DDF program also classifies them as good fats. Brown rice with vegetables and avocado is also a good lunch or dinner option.

As you begin following DDF, you might find that you are sensitive to brown rice and experience increased blood glucose numbers until your body understands your new way of fueling; however, for some brown rice may never work, and you might do better with quinoa or wild rice. Remember, it is all about bio-individuality. Experiment and discover what your body has to say about your choice.

A typical DDF week of fueling looks like this (snacks are optional):

Monday

Breakfast: one banana drizzled with tahini, coffee or tea (fruit + a seed butter)

Snack: a packet of almonds

Lunch: lettuce wraps—two romaine leaves with tuna fish and tomatoes (vegetable + protein)

Snack: a packet of almonds

Dinner: grilled turkey burgers with sautéed asparagus and a tossed salad with Brianna's French Vinaigrette dressing (protein + vegetable)

Beverages: unsweetened iced tea, hot tea, or water

Tuesday

Breakfast: two boiled eggs, coffee or tea (protein)

Snack: two stalks of celery with almond butter (vegetable + protein)

Lunch: turkey chili with a tossed salad (protein + vegetables)

Snack: a packet of almonds

Dinner: grilled salmon, steamed broccoli, and a tossed salad (protein + vegetables)

Beverages: unsweetened iced tea, hot tea, or water

Wednesday (meatless day)

Breakfast: an apple cut up with almond butter or sunflower seed butter, coffee or tea (fruit + nut/seed butter)

Snack: cup of vegetable broth (vegetable)

Lunch: baked sweet potato with half a can of black beans and an arugula salad with fresh sweet lemon (carb/starch + plant-based protein + vegetable)

Snack: a packet of almonds

Dinner: falafel with hummus and a small salad (plant-based protein + vegetables)

Beverages: unsweetened iced tea, hot tea, or water

Thursday

Breakfast: scrambled eggs with turkey sausages, coffee or tea (protein)

Snack: low-salt tomato or V8 juice with a stalk of celery (vegetable)

Lunch: white bean soup or vegetarian chili with side salad (plant-based protein + vegetables)

Snack: edamame

Dinner: brown rice pasta with mushroom Bolognese and a small salad (carb + vegetables)

Beverages: unsweetened iced tea, hot tea, or water

Friday (meatless day)

Breakfast: sprouted-grain English muffins with mashed avocado and sliced radishes, coffee or tea (carb/starch + vegetable) (Avocados are technically considered a single-seeded berry [fruit]; however, nutritionally, they are more like a vegetable and a good fat and are listed as such on USDA sites.)

Snack: coconut milk yogurt (nondairy) with sliced almonds

Lunch: lentil soup and small salad (protein + vegetables)

Snack: mixed berries with almond butter

Dinner: stir-fried vegetables with tofu and brown rice (vegetables + plant-based protein + carb/starch)

Beverages: unsweetened iced tea, hot tea, or water

Saturday

Breakfast: egg-white veggie omelet with sliced avocado, coffee or tea (protein + vegetable)

Lunch: fajitas (chicken, shrimp); substitute romaine leaves for tortillas (protein + vegetables)

Snack: pear with sunflower seed butter

Dinner: grilled chicken with sautéed zucchini and small salad (protein + vegetables)

Beverages: glass of wine followed by a glass of unsweetened iced tea or water, hot tea, or coffee

Sunday

Breakfast: shakshouka, coffee or tea (protein + vegetables)

Lunch: Caesar salad with grilled shrimp and dressing on the side (vegetables + protein)

Snack: half an avocado with sliced almonds

Dinner: cioppino with an arugula salad (protein + vegetables)

Beverages: Unsweetened iced tea, hot tea, or water

Before you set out for the grocery store, think about what your breakfasts, lunches, dinners, and snacks will look like. What will you drink during the week? If you want cream in your decaffeinated or regular coffee, will it be soy or coconut creamer, or have you decided that you can't give up your half and half (if so, use it sparingly)?

Be aware: Some medications have hypoglycemia (low blood sugar) as a side effect. So if you are eating to keep your blood glucose between 70 and 100 mg/dL, and then you take a medication that lowers your blood glucose, what do you think might happen? Your blood glucose could go below 70 mg/dL, so be vigilant about preventing that result! Always carry a healthy snack just in case. Make sure you are in contact with your physician and inform him or her about your commitment to DDF.

Please remember to begin each meal with a short, silent prayer of gratitude and love. Reflect on what it took to get that meal onto your plate. From the farmers who planted the seeds to those who harvested the fruits and vegetables, to the animals and fish who gave their lives, to those individuals who transported and packaged the food, along with store or restaurant employees and your culinary expertise—appreciate it all. Honor them and yourself by fueling your body according to its needs, not your desires. Nourishing your body is a sacred act of love.

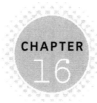

Meal Choices

"Put your future in good hands—your own."
—UNKNOWN

Menu Planning

Beverages

Decaf coffee

Unsweetened ice or hot tea

Hot water with lemon

Flat or sparkling water

Breakfast Choices

These are just examples:

Avocado toast

Bowl of berries with a heaping tablespoon or two of a nut or seed butter (almond, cashew, or sunflower)

Egg-white omelet with spinach, sun-dried tomatoes, and Daiya mozzarella cheese

Old-fashioned oatmeal (not one-minute, instant, or microwave—they are highly processed) with one teaspoon of cinnamon sprinkled on top and unsweetened almond milk (75 percent of my clients are unable to tolerate this breakfast due to glucose spike)

One banana (not a super-ripe one because it tends to be sweeter) with nut or seed butter

One apple cut up with nut or seed butter

Egg-white omelet with veggies* and nondairy cheese

Eggplant shakshuka

Scrambled eggs with sautéed veggies*

Grape Nuts, Grape Nut Flakes, or Uncle Sam's cereal with unsweetened almond milk (60 percent of my clients are unable to tolerate this breakfast)

Two boiled eggs alone or with veggies* or a salad

Turkey or chicken breakfast sausage with scrambled egg whites

Hemp bagel or sprouted-grain bagel with nondairy cream cheese or almond butter

Smoked salmon (lox) spread with nondairy cream cheese and rolled up

Smoothie

Tofu scramble with veggies

Zucchini frittata

Two Romaine leaves filled with scrambled eggs

*Broccoli, peppers, asparagus, zucchini, kale, spinach, tomatoes; no cooked carrots or cooked corn

Lunch Choices

Salad (prewashed, packaged salad provides up to four servings) with any kind of fish or chicken on top

Polenta squares with a salad

Soup (noncreamy, no noodles). You can purchase premade soups at a local health-conscious restaurant. Panera has a garden vegetable and a black bean soup. Serve with a side salad or coleslaw (get a bag of prechopped coleslaw and add onion powder and garlic powder, season with sea salt and pepper, sprinkle red wine vinegar or apple cider vinegar, and drizzle olive oil on top).

Arugula and fennel salad

Brussels sprout and fennel slaw

Lettuce wraps. Rinse romaine leaves; stir-fry onion, peppers, mushrooms, and pea pods in a small amount (one teaspoon) of sesame oil; season with tamari if desired; add leftover chicken, shrimp, tempeh, tofu, or beans; and place a generous spoonful on the leaf and roll up.

Kale with cannellini beans

Wedge. Cut a generous wedge from a head of lettuce, rinse, and place on a plate with tomatoes, cucumbers, and hard-boiled egg slices or one-third cup black beans; use your favorite dressing as long as it isn't high in sugar. I recommend Brianna's Real French Vinaigrette, as it has zero sugar.

Fajitas without the tortilla or, if you must, a flax seed tortilla

Half a bag of broccoli slaw mixed with one-third of a can of black beans and dressing

Vegetarian or turkey chili with a side salad

Salmon burger or turkey burger (grilled) with Dijon mustard with a side salad

Flax seed tortilla spread with hummus, chopped tomatoes, cucumbers, and/or other veggies, rolled up and sliced

Omelet with a salad

Romaine leaves with slices of turkey, mustard, tomatoes or filled with egg salad or tuna salad

Seaweed paper salad wraps

Snack Choices

Celery stalks with hummus, guacamole, or tuna

Crispy brussels sprouts

Unsalted tortilla chips with guacamole

Ten to twelve almonds or walnuts (unsalted)

Low-salt tomato or V8 juice with celery stalk or asparagus

Apple with almond butter

Pear with almond butter

Half an avocado sprinkled with sliced almonds

Boiled egg with mustard

Cup of vegetable or chicken broth

Coconut milk yogurt (nondairy) with slivered almonds

Bobo's Bar (original or almond)

Pickled vegetables: asparagus, cauliflower, green beans, okra, radishes, or zucchini

Keep packets of almonds in your car, briefcase, or purse to avoid low blood sugar. You should avoid becoming light-headed, which could lead to fainting, and you don't want to become ravenous from low blood sugar, which could cause inappropriate food choices.

Dinner Choices

Pan-seared salmon or halibut with caper relish

Grilled turkey or chicken sausages with sautéed sauerkraut

Tempeh or tofu veggie stir-fry

Brown rice pasta with marinara, pesto, or eggplant sauce

Quinoa salad

Stuffed cabbage rolls (no rice) with ground turkey and shredded zucchini

Zucchini lasagna

White bean soup and salad

Baked peppers stuffed with ground turkey or quinoa

Grilled salmon, salad, and steamed asparagus or broccoli

Bean and avocado salad

Mushroom Bolognese with brown rice pasta and salad

Veggie burger or salmon burger with sautéed red cabbage

Broccoli slaw with shrimp and Organicville Miso Ginger Vinaigrette

Roasted chicken and salad

Grape leaves stuffed with bulgur wheat or quinoa

Falafel with salad

Lima bean and zucchini stew

Turkey or vegetarian chili

Fish stew (cioppino)

Miso-glazed sea bass with roasted asparagus and mashed cauliflower

Baked chicken breasts with lemon and oregano and a salad

Omelet and salad

Burrito with veggies and beans, no rice

Brown rice and sautéed veggies

Brown rice mac and cheese (nondairy cheddar) and salad

Lentil soup and salad

Black bean posole

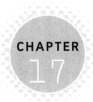

The Importance of Journaling and Meal Discovery Cards

Journaling is essential. It creates a road map to your destination of improved health, well-being, and weight loss. Journaling helps maintain accountability. It keeps you honest and will enable you to track your fueling (your meals and snacks), movement, and stress management.

The foundation of Data-Driven Fueling is intimate acquaintance with your body and your bio-individuality. Discovering the connection between your food choices, lifestyle, and stress level and the impact they have on blood glucose is essential to achieving your weight and health goals. Journaling provides insight and clarity. It showcases life choices, stressors, a view of progress, and increased knowledge and awareness.

I am all about data. Data-Driven Fueling is about collecting, organizing, and processing raw facts so that you can create information about yourself.

Although there are many diet, exercise, and diabetes apps you can download on your cell phone, they cannot replace old-fashioned journaling. Please feel free to use those to input what you eat, your stress level, and your activity/exercise; however, until the Forget Dieting! app becomes available, you should use the *Forget Dieting!* Journal. Writing about what you ate, how you felt during the day, your movement/exercise, and what worked or didn't work for you will have an impact on your thinking and behavior. It is a critical component in changing long-standing behaviors. You need the journal at your bedside, and you need to write down your daily behavior so that you can see patterns—good ones and bad ones. The goal is to Forget Dieting! and develop a lifestyle of Data-Driven Fueling.

In the beginning, you may feel like journaling is tedious and a waste of time. Change is not easy, but the first step to improved health and weight loss is to understand your body and how it processes what you eat and drink. Journaling provides that insight.

Journaling keeps things "real." There is no point in lying about what you ate, how much you exercised, or what your blood glucose numbers or tuning-in feelings were on a given day.

If you are honest in your journaling, commit to testing or tuning in, and record your data daily, you will see patterns emerge. Reviewing one week before the start of the next will aid you in your transformation. Listen to and learn from your body.

With a healthy, personalized diet, active lifestyle, and investment in stress management and holistic personal care, you will provide your body with tools that enable it to lose weight and heal.

If you choose to use a notebook, then please journal the following every day:

Date_____ Weight_____

Morning blood glucose_____ or tune-in feelings_____

Cup of hot water ____ yes ____ no

Breakfast _____ Time_____ Time + 90 minutes: glucose_____ Tune in feelings_____

Snack_____ Time_____ Time + 90 minutes: glucose_____ Tune in feelings_____

Lunch_____ Time_____ Time + 90 minutes:
glucose_____ Tune in feelings_____

Snack_____ Time_____ Time + 90 minutes:
glucose_____ Tune in feelings_____

Dinner_____ Time_____ Time + 90 minutes:
glucose_____ Tune in feelings_____

Stress level: (low) 1 2 3 4 5 6 7 8 9 10 (high)

Exercise ____ Yes ____ No Type _____

Meditation/deep breathing ____ Yes ____ No

Vitamins ____ Yes ____ No

Eight glasses of water ____ Yes ____ No

Observations _____

Meal Discovery Cards

Meal discovery cards are quick tools to help in your meal planning. By listing the date, what you ate, when you ate (breakfast, lunch, dinner, or snack), your blood glucose or tune-in before the meal, your blood glucose or tune-in ninety minutes after the meal, the source of the food (home cooked, take-out, or restaurant), and what you drank, the cards record what works for you and what doesn't. It takes the guesswork out of fueling.

Purchase index cards, a recipe/index card box, a green magic marker, and a red magic marker. Divide the box in half. The front half will be reserved for foods/meals that work for you. Divide that half into sections: breakfast, lunch, dinner, and snacks. The back half will be for cards that showcase foods/meals that didn't work for you and should also be divided into breakfast, lunch, dinner, and snacks. Fill out the card with the details, and then take either a green or a red marker and highlight the top right corner of the card. Green obviously indicates a good meal choice and red a bad one. A meal that raises your blood glucose should be avoided or saved for a splurge day.

The cards should look like this:

Date: _____ Testing: _____ Tuning in: _____

Breakfast: _____ Lunch: _____ Dinner: _____ Snack: _____

Home cooked: _____ Restaurant: _____

Name of restaurant: _____

Prepared food/grab and go: _____ Vendor: _____
_____

Meal: _____
_____
_____

Beverages: _____

Blood glucose #: _____ Tuning in*: _____
_____

Pancreas friendly: Yes _____ No _____

If no, a better choice would have been _____
_____
_____
_____

* If tuning in, describe physical feelings ninety minutes after eating.

An example of a **GOOD** DDF meal:

Date: <u>6/13/18</u> Testing: <u>X</u> Tuning in: _____

Breakfast: <u>X</u> Lunch: _____ Dinner: _____ Snack: _____

Home cooked: _____ Restaurant: <u>X</u>

Name of restaurant: <u>Oceanview</u>

Prepared food/grab and go: _____ Vendor: _____

Meal: <u>egg-white omelet with zucchini, asparagus, grilled onions, and tomatoes, side order of turkey sausage</u>

Beverages: <u>decaf coffee with soy milk and a glass of water</u>

Blood glucose #: <u>96</u> Tuning in*: _____

Pancreas friendly: Yes <u>X</u> No _____

If no, a better choice would have been _____

---

* If tuning in, describe physical feelings ninety minutes after eating.

Date: <u>6/13/18</u> Testing: _____ Tuning in: <u>X</u>

Breakfast: <u>X</u> Lunch: _____ Dinner: _____ Snack: _____

Home cooked: ____ Restaurant: <u>X</u>

Name of restaurant: <u>Oceanview</u>

Prepared food/grab and go: ____ Vendor: _____

Meal: <u>egg-white omelet with zucchini, asparagus, grilled onions and tomatoes, side order of turkey sausage</u>

Beverages: <u>decaf coffee with soy milk and a glass of water</u>

Blood glucose #: _____ Tuning in*: <u>no feelings of hunger or sleepiness. Feel great, just a bit thirsty</u>

Pancreas friendly: Yes <u>X</u> No _____

If no, a better choice would have been _____

---

* If tuning in, describe physical feelings ninety minutes after eating.

An example of a **BAD** DDF meal:

Date: <u>6/14/18</u> Testing: <u>X</u> Tuning in: _____

Breakfast: <u>X</u> Lunch: _____ Dinner: _____ Snack: _____

Home cooked: _____ Restaurant: <u>X</u>

Name of restaurant: <u>Snookies</u>

Prepared food/grab and go: _____ Vendor: _____

Meal: <u>Huevos rancheros with beans, rice, cheese, and tortilla with chips and salsa:</u>

Beverages: <u>coffee, cream, sugar</u>

Blood glucose #: <u>149</u> Tuning in*: _____

Pancreas friendly: Yes ____ No <u>X</u>

If no, a better choice would have been <u>huevos rancheros, no rice, no cheese, no tortilla, and no sugar or sugar substitute in my coffee</u>

* If tuning in, describe physical feelings ninety minutes after eating.

Date: <u>6/14/18</u> Testing: _____ Tuning in: <u>X</u>

Breakfast: <u>X</u> Lunch: _____ Dinner: _____ Snack: _____

Home cooked: _____ Restaurant: <u>X</u>

Name of restaurant: <u>Snookies</u>

Prepared food/grab and go: _____ Vendor: _____

Meal: <u>Huevos rancheros with beans, rice, cheese, and tortilla with chips and salsa</u>

Beverages: <u>coffee, cream, sugar</u>

Blood glucose #: _____ Tuning in*: <u>felt shaky, very hungry—wanted to stuff my mouth with anything after eating</u>

Pancreas friendly: Yes ___ No <u>X</u>

If no, a better choice would have been <u>huevos rancheros, no rice, no cheese, no tortilla, and no sugar or sugar substitute in my coffee</u>

* If tuning in, describe physical feelings ninety minutes after eating.

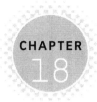

What to Do with a High Glucose Number

"If there is no struggle, there is no progress."

—FREDERICK DOUGLASS

I've had many experiences with high glucose numbers after a poor meal choice or unbelievable stress. I'll give you a couple of examples. One day I went to pick up my father's prescription at the pharmacy. As I waited in line to check out, I saw a pack of chocolate-covered pretzel M&Ms, prominently advertised as having only one hundred calories. I thought, *Hmmm, one hundred calories. If I were on a twelve-hundred-calorie diet, I would consider fitting that into my day's allotment.* I decided to purchase the M&Ms and see what my body had to say about my choice. When I got to my car, I retrieved my glucometer and tested my blood glucose. It was under 90 mg/dL. I ate the bag of M&Ms and set my phone alarm for ninety minutes. I tested again, and my blood sugar was over 130 mg/dL!

Another day I lunched with my husband at a Mexican restaurant. I know that chicken or shrimp fajitas without tortillas along with unsweetened iced tea works for me; however, I was feeling sad. My precious father had passed away seven weeks prior, and I decided to give in to my blue feelings. I ordered unsweetened iced tea (a plus), but then I ordered chicken fajitas and piled them onto two tortillas. In addition, I had chips with salsa. My blood glucose prior to lunch was 79 mg/dL. By the time I returned home, I felt sleepy, and my mind was foggy. I decided to check my glucose after ninety minutes. It was at 132 mg/dL! Up forty-two points. This was a form of self-sabotage.

I know my body very well, and so will you as you plug into the DDF lifestyle. I understand what fuel works for and against my body. I don't have to test very often now, but I do tune in. The other night my husband and I went out to dinner with friends. I don't eat red meat very often (approximately four to five times a year), but at that meal I wanted to have a small steak. I ordered a dinner salad and the steak and substituted spinach for the potato. But I did something that I knew would affect my glucose and my weight: I had two pieces of focaccia while I waited for my salad. I didn't need to test. I didn't feel great after the meal. The next morning my body continued its conversation with me. I got on the scale, and I was up two pounds. I did not practice proper food combining, and my body let me know. That day I practiced what I preach: I went on a liquid fast. I also went for a long walk with my dog. My body needed a break, and it needed to use up the excess fuel. The next day when I got on the scale, I had lost the two pounds I had gained the day before.

There are several reasons for this result: the meal was at a restaurant (restaurants are notorious for using more salt than anyone would use at home); mild dehydration could have been a factor, which can cause the body to retain fluids; and I loaded up with focaccia and didn't follow the basics of proper food combining (improper food combining can lead to both increased fat storage and water retention; for every gram of carbohydrate you store as glycogen, your tissues must retain three grams of water).

The number on the scale measures fat along with bone, fluids, muscle, organs, connective tissue, and any food you've yet to digest. If you haven't effectively emptied your bowels (which can cause bloating), it can show up on the scale.

Whether it has been caused by a stressful situation, indulgence in "calorie-friendly" snacks, or improper food combining, you can counteract a glucose dump with movement/exercise or a liquid fast to return to normal glucose levels.

If you test and discover that your glucose has spiked more than thirty points, you need to deal with it! Use up that excess glucose before it has a chance to get stored in fat cells.

How do you utilize the excess glucose before the body has a chance to store it? I'll give you examples. After I ate the fajitas with the tortillas along with salsa and chips and tested my blood glucose ninety minutes after the meal (with a reading of 142 mg/dL), I picked up my hula hoop. I had to use up that excess fuel. I jacked up the music and hula hooped to two songs, and then I tested. My blood glucose had gone down to 82 mg/dL. Again, my body responded. It used the excess (unnecessary) fuel.

Now I don't want you to think that you can abuse your body and your pancreas by eating whatever you want and then negating that poor choice with hula hooping or another form of movement.

By embracing DDF as your lifestyle, think how you might improve your health and reduce your weight even more by incorporating an evening stroll after dinner like people in so many other cultures (Spain, Italy, Greece).

Nobody is perfect. There will be slip-ups. The good news is that there is a way to correct them. Having fewer slip-ups is the goal of adhering to the Data-Driven Fueling lifestyle. Preventing slip-ups is what you are working toward. However, never berate yourself or feel defeated. You can turn a negative into a positive. Your new lifestyle is not going to happen overnight. You and your body have started a dialogue that is long overdue. You have so much to share and so many goals to work toward! It's a magical partnership.

Vitamins

"If you aren't going all the way, why go at all?"

—JOE NAMATH

I am always asked about what vitamins I take. Each and every one of us has different needs, so I will address what I feel are the basic ones for adults ages twenty-one and older. You may supplement with other vitamins according to your deficiencies; however, always speak with your physician because certain supplements/vitamins can interfere with prescription medication.

I recommend the following vitamins to promote a healthy heart and pancreas. Taking these vitamins, accompanied by Data-Driven Fueling and exercise, should be part of your way of life. Always check the labels for recommended dosages and *do not exceed* them. Higher doses will not speed up weight loss! Take vitamins with a meal.

Vitamin Supplements

The doses are based on the needs of and recommended daily allowance for the average adult. Remember, it is always best to receive vitamins through organic food sources; however, this is difficult in today's world, so supplementation is often necessary.

A landmark study by Donald Davis and his team of researchers at the University of Texas at Austin's Department of Chemistry and Biochemistry (published in December 2004) in the *Journal of the American College of Nutrition* found reliable decline in the amount of protein, calcium, phosphorus, iron, riboflavin (vitamin B2), and vitamin C in forty-three different vegetable and fruits over the past half century. Davis and his colleagues studied the U.S. Department of Agriculture's nutritional data from both 1950 and 1999. Their conclusion: The decline in nutritional content is due to the preponderance of agricultural practices designed to improve traits (size, growth rate, pest resistance) other than nutrition. When possible grow your own, buy organic, and/or shop at your local farmer's market.

The following vitamins I have recommended for adults in addition to a healthy diet:

- One multivitamin
- Super B complex
- Vitamin C (1,000 mg)
- Vitamin D (2000 IU) twice a day (a.m. and p.m.)
- A calcium, magnesium, and zinc combination (taken at bedtime)
- Coenzyme Q10 (200 mg). CoQ10 has been noted to promote heart health; however, it can also decrease your response to Coumadin (check with your physician).
- Fish oil. I prefer the liquid (Carlson's), one to two teaspoons per day. Make sure that the omega-3 fatty acids include high levels of EPA and DHA (800 mg EPA and 500 mg DHA would be the total for the day).

- Tart cherry concentrate (800 mg), twice a day (a.m. and p.m.). Tart cherry juice is known to reduce inflammation in the joints. It helps me. You can also purchase Montmorency Tart Cherry Juice concentrate and mix two ounces with four ounces of water. Drink it twice a day.

If I feel a cold or flu coming on, I take 3,000 mg of garlic and 3,000 mg of vitamin C immediately; then I take 1,000–2,000 mg of each three times a day and gargle with warm saltwater until the symptoms subside.

In addition to taking my vitamins, I "pound" on my sternum (chest bone) when I'm in the shower in order to stimulate my thymus. The thymus gland has a right and a left lobe. It is located between your lungs, behind your sternum.

The thymus shrinks as you get older. At birth, the thymus is about 4–6 centimeters long, 2.5–5 centimeters wide, and 1 centimeter thick and weighs about one ounce. It is small but amazing! It reaches its maximum size during adolescence, and as you age it shrinks and is replaced by fat tissue.

The thymus is a small incubator and warehouse. It provides an area for lymphocytes to mature into T cells (T lymphocytes). Lymphocytes are produced by the bone marrow and then travel to the thymus to mature into T cells and wait for a call to duty. These T cells are on high alert to fight infection, foreign substances, and disease in your body.

In addition to providing warrior cells, the thymus makes hormones (thymosin) that assist in T cell development and production and regulate the immune system. Once T cells mature, they are released into the bloodstream to aid the immune system in its battle against disease. Not all T cells circulate in the bloodstream. Many are sent to the lymph nodes and spleen to continue maturation and serve as backup when needed by the body. By the time you reach adolescence, the thymus has produced the T cells needed by your living machine.

Many holistic practitioners and eastern medicine gurus believe that thymus shrinkage after puberty has to do with lack of thymus stimulation. What happens to anything that isn't stimulated or is neglected?

The next time you're in the shower, think Johnny Weissmuller (the original Tarzan), beat on your chest (actually your sternum/breast bone) with the tips of your index, middle, ring, and baby fingers (doesn't matter which hand) or your fist, open your mouth, and give the Tarzan yell (for about fifteen to twenty seconds). For those of you too young to remember Johnny Weissmuller, just go to YouTube and search for "Johnny Weissmuller Tarzan Call." This simple maneuver will strengthen your immune system, increase your life-force energy, release fear, and increase strength and vitality. FYI: Researchers at major medical centers are currently working in labs to create medications that will stimulate the thymus. Why take a pill when all you have to do is beat on your chest?

Food Sources of Vitamins

- Mixed carotenoids—pumpkin, sweet potatoes, carrots, butternut squash, tuna, cantaloupe, mangoes, broccoli, apricots, and watermelon
- Vitamin A—cod liver oil, egg yolks, butter, raw whole milk, liver
- Folic acid—legumes, poultry, tuna, wheat germ, mushrooms, oranges, asparagus, broccoli, strawberries, cantaloupes, bananas, spinach
- Vitamin B6—fish, avocados, lima beans, soybeans, chicken, bananas, cauliflower, green peppers, potatoes, raisins, spinach
- Vitamin B1—pork, wheat germ, pasta, peanuts, legumes, watermelon, brown rice, oranges, oatmeal, eggs
- Vitamin B2—milk, cottage cheese, avocados, tangerines, prunes, asparagus, broccoli, beef, salmon, turkey, mushrooms
- Vitamin B3—meats, poultry, fish, peanut butter, legumes, soybeans, whole grains, broccoli, baked potatoes, asparagus

- Vitamin B12—salmon, eggs, cheese, swordfish, tuna, clams, mussels, oysters
- Panthothenic acid—fish, whole grains, mushrooms, avocados, broccoli, peanuts, cashews, lentils, soybeans, eggs
- Biotin—oatmeal, nuts, eggs, wheat germ, poultry, cauliflower, legumes
- Vitamin C—citrus fruit, strawberries, tomatoes, bell peppers, spinach, cabbage, melon, broccoli, raspberries, kiwi fruit
- Vitamin D—sunlight, butter, tuna, milk, eggs, salmon
- Vitamin E—nut and vegetable oils, wheat germ, mangoes, blackberries, broccoli, apples, spinach, whole wheat, peanuts
- Vitamin K—tomatoes, eggs, dairy products, carrots, avocados, spinach, broccoli, cabbage, brussels sprouts, parsley
- Calcium—kale, turnip greens, almonds, green beans, milk, cheese, yogurt, salmon, sardines with bones, broccoli
- Magnesium—molasses, spinach, wheat germ, nuts, pumpkin seeds, seafood, baked potatoes, broccoli, bananas
- Selenium—meats, whole grains, dairy products, fish, shellfish, mushrooms, Brazil nuts
- Potassium—potatoes, avocados, bananas, yogurt, cantaloupe, milk, mushrooms, tomatoes, spinach
- Zinc—lean beef, seafood, lima beans, legumes, nuts, poultry, dairy products

Sodium is also important; however, you probably get more than enough in your regular diet.

What to Do If
You Hit a Plateau

"Happiness is the feeling you're feeling
when you want to keep feeling it."

—AUTHOR UNKNOWN

"All or nothing" thinking makes everything more difficult, especially losing weight. Do not focus on losing fifty pounds. Instead, break it down and strive for two pounds per week. If faced with a huge rock, would you try to pick up the whole thing or chip away at it until you were able to remove it? Be mindful that all good things come to those who have patience and an understanding of their organic machine.

I've heard too many times, "I lost twenty-five pounds and just couldn't lose anymore!" "I gave up. I was starving myself, working out like a fiend, and only lost twenty pounds." These clients gave it their all, stopped losing weight, became frustrated, and just quit. The results weren't worth the sacrifice.

Our bodies are hardwired to survive. The body stops losing weight because it believes you are in danger. It may believe you are experiencing famine, and it is going to hold on to every fat gram in your tummy, thighs, upper arms, butt, and face because it believes you need them.

This idea especially applies if you've been having a party at every meal and then the party is over. The body doesn't understand that you have made a mindful decision about what to put in your mouth. It simply registers that you no longer have access to that bounty you've been stuffing yourself with before. So it is going to hold tight to the fat to make sure you survive.

> *To overcome this stagnation, implement the "plateau buster" plan. The plateau buster is only used if you have not lost a pound in seven days. The plateau buster reboots your body from famine to weight-loss thinking. Pick one protein out of these three: chicken, fish, or tofu. Now pick one vegetable out of these three: broccoli, asparagus, or zucchini.*

Whichever protein and vegetable you pick (for example, fish and asparagus), you must eat just that for each meal for three days. I don't care whether you grill the fish, bake it, or sauté it, but use the same kind of fish each time. The vegetable can be steamed, sautéed, or eaten raw, but it should be the same vegetable each time. For example, if you decided to eat salmon and asparagus, then you would eat salmon and asparagus for breakfast, lunch, and dinner for three days. After three days, you would resume your Data-Driven Fueling lifestyle.

During the three days of plateau busting, increase your activity a notch. Walk or bike an extra few blocks or a mile. Hula hoop to a third song; do seventy-five jumping jacks instead of fifty; whatever you are doing for exercise, increase it during this time.

In addition, I have used Super Dieter's Tea or Smooth Move Tea during this plateau period. I will drink a strong cup before going to bed with the understanding that I don't have to be anywhere before noon the next day (because you want to be near a bathroom). There is nothing more uncomfortable than being in a meeting or on an airplane after drinking the tea the night before. Many of my clients use these teas once a month. Cleansing your gastrointestinal tract on a monthly basis can't hurt you.

Every time you reach a plateau (i.e., haven't lost a pound in seven days), eat according to the plateau buster. My clients who have to lose eighty or one hundred pounds utilize the plateau buster after approximately every twenty to twenty-five pounds lost. Why? Because that twenty-pound loss seems to scare the body, and it won't give up even a quarter of a pound. This is one of the reasons why most diets fail. The dieter becomes frustrated and gives up. Don't ever give up. You and your body are in a partnership, and it is only looking out for you. The plateau buster will guide it into your next phase of weight loss.

Eating Out of Your Element: College and Travel

"You measure the size of the accomplishment by the obstacles you had to overcome to reach your goals."

—BOOKER T. WASHINGTON

College

College and travel can present problems for those who are trying to lose weight or live a healthy lifestyle. I've discovered, however, that absence from home can actually aid in the effort to lose weight and improve health and well-being. The Data-Driven Fueling lifestyle is actually much easier to maintain when you are not at home. Wish I had figured this out forty years ago.

When I went away to nursing school and walked into the cafeteria for the first time, I was beyond excited! I said to my roommate, "You mean I can pick out whatever I want, and it is covered on the meal plan?" She answered, "Yep!" Well, I ate my way up about twenty pounds, and so did most of my friends. We thought we would counter that by joining Elaine Powers. We would go to that "exercise" facility and place our backsides, thighs, and upper arms on wooden rollers. We never changed our cafeteria selections and weekend pizza parties or stopped drinking beer. We were at a loss as to why we did not lose a pound.

College-bound students, especially females, are often warned about gaining the "freshman fifteen." The cause of this common weight gain situation is multifaceted. The cafeteria offers a tempting assortment of desserts, pastas, burgers, and fries. Couple that with late-night pizzas ordered to the dorm, alcohol consumption, and drugs. Beer is calorically dense. Marijuana use stimulates the munchies. Stress, due to being away from home, dealing with roommate situations, preparing homework, and studying for exams, also contributes to weight gain. All these factors add to the numbers on the scale.

Data-Driven Fueling Suggestions for Eating at College

- *Breakfast in your dorm room:* Eat an apple, pear, or banana served with nuts or topped with a nut or seed butter.
- *Breakfast in the cafeteria:* Avoid waffles, pancakes, bagels, and French toast. Choose eggs (omelet, over easy, or hard-boiled) alone or with turkey or chicken sausages. Or you could skip the sausages and add a salad. Another breakfast choice: a smoothie with fruit, spinach, kale, and protein powder.
- *Lunch:* Eat a salad and a protein (chicken, fish, turkey, beans, or hard-boiled eggs). Avoid combining carbs (rice, pasta, or potatoes) with protein. Avoid desserts; enjoy a dessert at only one meal per week. Trust me, you will enjoy and appreciate that dessert much more than if you were eating sweets every day.

- *Dinner:* This meal will be essentially the same as lunch: salad, protein, and veggies. Remember, you can still enjoy going out with friends. Pick one day out of the week (Friday or Saturday night) to enjoy pizza with friends (but add a huge salad to complement it). If your friends suggest Mexican food, go! You can enjoy fajitas without the tortillas and tortilla chips with guacamole instead of salsa (chips and salsa alone will spike glucose; guacamole has a fat content that does not usually spike glucose). Avoid margaritas (high sugar content). Follow every alcoholic beverage with a glass or bottle of water.

Travel

My family never went on vacations, and we rarely ate out. We couldn't afford to. My dad's two-week vacations might include a trip to the zoo or a museum, but mostly it was time for him to work on projects around the house. When I graduated from nursing school and went with a friend to Fort Lauderdale, I was a girl gone *wild* at the restaurants. Breakfast might be 2 × 2 × 2 (two pancakes, two eggs, two sausages), followed by a lunch of a burger and fries; dinner would be a steak and a baked potato (with sour cream and butter) or pasta with meat sauce and lots of bread and butter. My concept of vacation travel was an open invitation to gluttony. Screw it, I was on vacation, and I deserved to treat myself for working so hard. When I returned from a vacation, I often brought back not only souvenirs but also five-plus pounds. What a joke! I wasn't treating myself; I was abusing myself.

Travel—be it a weekend in Vegas, a cruise, or a week in Italy—does not have to expand your waistline. You can keep your weight and health in check. When you dine out for every meal, you can expect water-weight gain because restaurants are notorious for preparing food with excess salt.

Since I began following the Data-Driven Fueling program and understanding how my body processes food, most of my travel results in weight loss (one to two pounds). How is this possible? Actually, I find maintaining my weight so much easier while traveling. I don't have access to my pantry or my kitchen to tempt me. Snacking is eliminated. I am always on the go. Whether traveling for work or vacation, I'm busy, without a lot of down time. I'm much more active. Sightseeing and exploring the wonders of your destination provide so much to do that you can't help but be on the move. It's difficult to be a couch potato watching TV when you are traveling. Take advantage of that.

Cruise ships are notorious for their buffets and culinary offerings, and yet they provide ample opportunities for movement/exercise, whether it's swimming in the pool, taking exercise classes, doing yoga, walking around the ship, or dancing the night away. There are no excuses to just sit and eat.

Data-Driven Fueling Suggestions for Eating While Traveling

- Always follow an alcoholic beverage with a glass of water or unsweetened iced tea before you have a second alcoholic drink. Or you can make a spritzer (half wine, half sparkling water), which cuts the sugar content of the wine, or drink vodka on ice.
- Maintain your DDF Calendar (e.g., Wednesdays and Fridays are meatless).
- I pack small packages of nuts for snacks, and I take along packets of almond butter to use on an apple, pear, or banana for breakfast or a snack. I also pack Bobo's Bars (original and almond).
- Lunch and dinner are usually a no-brainer: protein (whether animal or plant-based) along with a salad and veggies. During a one-week vacation—let's say a trip to Italy—I'll indulge in an occasional pasta dish or a slice of pizza. However, I will not eat that every day of my vacation, because it is bad for my pancreas, my health, and my weight.

- Practice proper food combining, especially with buffets.
- Remember, your mind may be in vacation mode, but your body never gets a vacation from processing what you eat and drink.
- Don't treat yourself with food; treat yourself with the purchase of something that will remind you of your travel experience. It will last longer than the memory of a meal.
- Ask that the chef go light on salt.
- Remember, whether you are home, traveling, or away at school, health issues (a cold or flu and even menstruation) will cause fluid retention, and you may gain a couple of pounds. Don't get frustrated. Keep to your DDF lifestyle, and when the issue has passed, you will shed those pounds of fluid.
- Always remember that once you have a strong foundation of DDF, no matter where you go, you will be OK. You know how to make the right choices. You know how to fuel your machine. Nothing can deter you from your healthy lifestyle.

Recipes for Meals and Liquid Fasts

Liquid Fast

Apple Cider Vinegar Cleanse/Fasting Drink

> 12 ounces water
>
> 4 tablespoons Bragg Apple Cider Vinegar
>
> 1 teaspoon ground cinnamon
>
> 3 tablespoons lemon juice
>
> 1 pinch cayenne pepper
>
> ½ tablespoon honey (raw if possible) [if it raises blood glucose, omit]

Simply mix and enjoy!

Green Juice

    1 green apple (cored and cut up)

    1 cup kale leaves (no stems)

    1 celery stalk (chopped)

    6 mint leaves (include stems)

    2 tablespoons lemon or lime juice (freshly squeezed)

    1 medium cucumber (cut up)

    1–2 cups fresh spinach

    ¾ cup water

Place all ingredients into a blender. Blend at the highest level to "liquefy." You may enjoy the green juice with pulp or pour through a strainer to remove pulp. Serves two.

Smoothie

    1 scoop Vega protein powder

    ½ cup blueberries or ½ apple, cut up

    ½ banana (I peel bananas, cut in half, and freeze the unused portion)

    1 cup kale or 2 leaves

    1 cup romaine or 2 leaves (feel free to mix it up with the following: romaine, kale, collard, Swiss chard, spinach, arugula)

    4–5 ice cubes

    1 cup unsweetened almond milk

Place all ingredients in a blender until smooth.

    Feel free to add avocado instead of banana and strawberries instead of blueberries; experiment with different fruits. Keep in mind that some fruits may significantly raise your blood glucose. It is important to rule out the "bad" ones by testing or tuning in.

Appetizers/Snacks

Polenta Squares

I love to serve these tasty squares with a large salad (no animal protein).

> 12 tablespoons yellow cornmeal
>
> 3 cups low-salt vegetable broth
>
> 1 cup Go Veggie Vegan Parmesan Cheese
>
> salt and pepper to taste

Whisk yellow and white cornmeal in a bowl to blend. Bring broth to boil in a medium saucepan on medium high heat. Slowly whisk in cornmeal. Reduce heat to low and continue to whisk until mixture boils and becomes thick (approximately five minutes). Remove from heat. Whisk in three-quarters of the Go Veggie Vegan Parmesan Cheese and season with a minimal amount of salt and pepper.

Pour polenta into an 8 × 8 × 2 baking pan; smooth the top. Cool until firm or chill overnight. Preheat broiler. Cut polenta into sixteen squares; brush with oil and arrange squares (oil side down) on a baking/cookie sheet. Brush top with oil and broil until golden brown (about three minutes) per side; then sprinkle with the remaining quarter cup of Parmesan cheese.

Crispy Brussels Sprouts

> 3–4 tablespoons extra virgin olive oil
>
> 1½ pounds brussels sprouts, trimmed and cut in half
>
> 1 teaspoon sea salt or kosher salt
>
> ½ cup pomegranate seeds

Preheat oven to 400°. Place rack in the upper third of the oven. Place brussels sprouts in a large bowl; add olive oil and salt. Mix gently and do not discard any leaves that fall off. Using tongs, place brussels sprouts cut side down on a baking sheet (including discarded leaves).

Bake for fifteen to twenty-five minutes. During this time, use tongs to turn them, and check on them frequently because the size of the sprouts will affect the cooking time. The outside of the sprouts should be moderately charred.

Remove from the oven, place on a serving tray, and sprinkle with pomegranate seeds.

Breakfast

Egg-White Omelet with Spinach, Sun-Dried Tomatoes, and Daiya Mozzarella Cheese

   3 egg whites, beaten, or ½ cup egg whites from a carton

   2 teaspoons butter or olive oil

   2 cups baby spinach

   ½–⅔ cup sun-dried tomatoes, chopped (sun-dried tomatoes packed in olive oil should be drained)

   ¼ cup Daiya Mozzarella Cheese (vegan)

   salt and pepper to taste

Use a small nonstick pan. Melt or heat half the butter or olive oil; add spinach and sauté until wilted. Remove from pan and place on a plate. Add the rest of the butter or olive oil to the pan (make sure it coats the whole pan) and pour in egg whites. Tilt the pan to spread the egg whites out; cook over medium heat until set. Arrange spinach, sun-dried tomatoes, and "cheese" on half the eggs; then gently lift the other side to fold over the filling. Place a cover on top, turn off the heat, and let sit for two minutes. Season with salt and pepper.

Eggplant Shakshuka

2 tablespoons olive oil

1 small onion, chopped (1 cup)

12 pitted Greek olives (green or black), cut in half

1½ teaspoons paprika

1½ teaspoons ground cumin

¼ teaspoon red pepper flakes

1 medium eggplant, cut into cubes

1½ cups crushed tomatoes (fresh or canned)

3 cloves garlic, minced

⅓ cup cilantro, chopped

¾ cup water

4 large eggs

salt and pepper to taste

Pour oil into medium (approximately ten-inch) nonstick skillet. Add onion, olives, eggplant, garlic, paprika, cumin, and red pepper flakes. Cook over medium heat, stirring occasionally until eggplant is tender. Add crushed tomatoes and water. Reduce heat to simmer. Cover and cook for ten to twelve minutes, stirring occasionally. Add half the cilantro. If sauce is too thick, add one to two tablespoons of water to thin. Season with salt and pepper.

Make four deep wells in the mixture with the back of a spoon. Crack and pour an egg into each well, spacing properly. Cover and continue to simmer for four to five minutes. Remove pan from heat and let stand covered for a minute or two (make sure egg whites are set). Uncover and sprinkle with remaining cilantro. Serves four.

Avocado Toast

1–2 slices sprouted-grain bread or 1 sprouted-grain English muffin

1 ripe (not overripe) avocado, cut, halved, and scooped out

salt and pepper to taste

Mash the avocado in a bowl, not on the bread or muffin. Season with sea salt or kosher salt to taste. Toast bread or muffin and spread with avocado.

There are so many variations on avocado toast. You can add sliced radishes or tomatoes; you can sprinkle the toast with cilantro, arugula, spinach, toasted sesame, or pumpkin seeds. I substitute vegan cream cheese for avocado sometimes and eat it with sliced tomatoes and arugula. Serves one.

Tofu Scramble

2 tablespoons olive oil

28 ounces tofu (extra firm)

1 small onion, thinly sliced

1 small red bell pepper, finely chopped

1 small green bell pepper, finely chopped

½ teaspoon ground coriander

½ teaspoon ground cumin

1½ teaspoons ground turmeric

1 package baby spinach

¼ cup fresh cilantro, chopped (optional)

kosher salt and freshly ground pepper to taste

10 cherry tomatoes, halved

sliced avocado

Place tofu on a plate lined with layers of paper towels, top with more paper towels, and place a heavy pot on top (to squeeze liquid out of the tofu) for ten minutes. Remove paper towels and break up tofu with a fork to resemble scrambled eggs.

Heat oil in a large pan over medium heat. Add onions, peppers, and spinach; stir occasionally and make sure moisture from the spinach has evaporated and onions and peppers are softened (three to four minutes). Stir in coriander and cumin. Cook one to two minutes. Stir in tofu, then turmeric. Stir, and then add cilantro and season with salt and pepper. Serve scrambled tofu with sliced avocados and tomatoes on top.

Lunch

Brussels Sprout and Fennel Slaw

2 cups brussels sprouts, thinly sliced (a mandolin is a great tool and makes slicing easier, but watch your fingers!)

2 cups fennel, thinly sliced

1–2 lemons, zested and juiced (depending on your taste; do you like your salads dressed lightly?)

2–4 tablespoons white balsamic vinegar (again, it depends on how much dressing you enjoy)

1–2 tablespoons olive oil or grapeseed oil

½ cup fresh parsley, chopped

1 clove garlic, minced

salt and pepper to taste

Whisk together in a bowl lemon zest and juice, oil, vinegar, and garlic. In a separate bowl, mix brussels sprouts, fennel, and parsley. Pour dressing over slaw and mix well. Salt and pepper to taste. Serves six to eight.

Kale with Cannellini Beans

1½ pounds kale or mixed greens (kale and collard), stems and ribs removed

1 small onion, finely diced

1½ tablespoons olive oil

2 plump garlic cloves, minced

1 pinch red pepper flakes

2 teaspoons rosemary, chopped

½ cup dry white wine

1⅓ cups cooked cannellini beans (rinse well if canned)

freshly grated Parmesan (optional; may use vegan Parmesan)

salt and pepper to taste

Simmer the kale in salted water until tender (seven to ten minutes). Drain, reserving the cooking water, and chop the leaves. In a large skillet, sauté the onion in the oil with the garlic, pepper flakes, and rosemary for about three minutes. Add the wine, stirring continually for three minutes. Add the beans, kale, and enough cooking water to keep the mixture loose. Heat through, taste for salt, season with pepper, and serve with a dusting of Parmesan.[1]

Quinoa Salad

1 cup arugula

½ avocado, sliced

2 artichoke hearts, cut in half

6 cherry tomatoes, cut in half

1 cup quinoa, rinsed

2 cups vegetable broth

lemon vinaigrette

⅓ cup canned chickpeas or cannellini beans, heated

Bring the vegetable broth to a boil. Stir in the quinoa, and then turn the heat down to low. Cover and simmer until all the liquid is absorbed (about fifteen minutes). Use a fork to fluff and separate the grains.

Line a bowl or dinner plate with the arugula. Slice avocado, tomatoes, and artichoke hearts. Spoon beans or chickpeas on top of the arugula. Ladle ¾ cup of the quinoa on top of the beans/chickpeas. Arrange avocados, tomatoes, and artichokes. Dress the salad lightly. Serves one.

Lemon Vinaigrette

⅔ cup olive oil

⅓ cup fresh lemon juice

sea salt or kosher salt, fresh ground pepper to taste

Whisk ingredients together. Save extra vinaigrette in a sealed container.

Simple Arugula and Fennel Salad

1 bag arugula

1 fennel bulb, shaved (use a mandolin) or sliced very thin

¼ cup pine nuts

juice from 2 lemons

sea salt or kosher salt

On medium heat, place pine nuts in a small pan and lightly toast. Place arugula in a large bowl, add fennel, drizzle lemon over salad, season with salt to taste, and top with pine nuts. Serves two as a main meal and four as a side salad.

Seaweed Salad Wrap

Miso Mayo

> 1 cup vegan mayonnaise
>
> ¼ cup miso
>
> 1 tablespoon lemon
>
> 1 tablespoon soy sauce or tamari

Place all ingredients in a bowl and blend well.

Wraps

> 1 cucumber sliced julienne style
>
> 1 tomato, chopped
>
> 1–2 romaine leaves, chopped
>
> handful of spinach
>
> 2 sheets nori seaweed

*Optional: May add a can of salmon or tuna (drained) to the wrap

Lay nori sheets on a cutting board. Spread miso mayo on sheet. At one end of a sheet, arrange your "salad" and roll the nori starting from the side with the salad. Repeat with the second nori sheet. May use extra sauce to dip your nori wrap in.

Dinner

Brown Rice Pasta with Pesto Sauce

> 16 ounces brown rice pasta
>
> vegan or regular pesto*

Vegan Pesto

> 2–3 large cloves garlic
>
> 1 large bunch basil (approximately three cups, loosely packed)
>
> 6 tablespoons raw pine nuts or walnuts (or a combination of the two)
>
> ¾–1 teaspoon salt, or to taste
>
> 6 tablespoons extra virgin olive oil
>
> ¼ cup nutritional yeast (optional) or vegan Parmesan cheese

Place garlic, salt, and pine nuts in a food processor and pulse until finely chopped. Add basil. Process until smooth, and then add olive oil, nutritional yeast, or Parmesan.

Cook pasta (follow directions on the box if available), drain, and place in a pasta bowl or back in the pot and fold in the pesto sauce. Serve with a salad. Serves four.

*When in a rush, it is much easier to use premade pesto available at your local grocery store.

Zucchini Lasagna

This is one of my favorite recipes.

> 3–4 large zucchinis, thinly sliced lengthwise (I use a mandolin because it is easier.)

2 cups vegetable broth

1 cup quinoa, rinsed and drained

½ cup tomato sauce

¼ cup onion, finely chopped

1 teaspoon dried oregano

¼ cup fresh basil leaves, chopped (I like to use kitchen scissors because it is easier.)

½ –1 teaspoon salt to taste

¼ cup fresh parsley leaves, chopped (Use the scissors.)

2 tablespoons nondairy cream cheese (I use Tofutti.)

25 ounces marinara sauce (I use Lucini's Organic Tuscan Marinara Sauce, which only has three grams of sugar, or you can use your own marinara sauce recipe.)

½–1 cup nondairy cheese, shredded (Daiya mozzarella)

Preheat your oven to 400°. Place zucchini slices on a couple of paper towels. Cover with more paper towels to drain moisture (I prefer not to use salt to draw the moisture out).

Bring vegetable broth, quinoa, onion, and oregano to a boil. Then add tomato sauce (not marinara sauce). Next add salt. Begin with half a teaspoon; stir and taste. Cover the pot and reduce heat to medium/low and simmer for twenty to twenty-five minutes, until the liquid is absorbed. Remove from heat, and stir in basil, parsley, and cream cheese.

Spoon ¼ cup of marinara sauce over the bottom of a 13 × 9 lasagna pan. Lay zucchini slices over the marinara sauce just as you would lasagna noodles. Spoon/spread half of quinoa mixture over the zucchini, and then pour one-third of the marinara sauce on top (spreading evenly) and sprinkle with shredded mozzarella. Repeat with more zucchini slices, the remaining quinoa, and one-third of the marinara sauce. Top with remaining zucchini slices, remaining marinara, and shredded cheese. Bake lasagna for thirty minutes or until the zucchini is tender and the cheese bubbles. Serves approximately six.

Pan-Seared Salmon or Halibut with Caper Relish

2 small shallots, thinly sliced (⅓ cup)

1 teaspoon sea salt

2 lemons, quartered

4 tablespoons capers

½ cup kalamata olives, drained and chopped

1 pint cherry tomatoes, cut in half

½ teaspoon red pepper flakes

⅓ cup extra virgin olive oil

¾ cup fresh basil, chopped

Salmon or Halibut

1½–2 pounds fish, cut into four pieces

½ teaspoon salt

½ teaspoon freshly ground black pepper

2 tablespoons extra virgin olive oil or butter

Slice the lemons into quarters and squeeze out the juice (removing seeds). Place the lemons and the juice in a bowl with the shallots and salt. Add capers, kalamata olives, pepper flakes, tomatoes, and ⅓ cup of olive oil. Cover bowl and set aside to marinate for at least four hours. (Making the relish the day before is preferable. Remember to refrigerate it, but take it out of the refrigerator at least one hour before cooking the fish.) Before you cook the fish, simmer the relish in a small pot. You will want to garnish the fish with warm, not cold, relish.

Sprinkle fish with salt and pepper. In a large nonstick skillet or cast-iron pan, heat the oil on medium-high until it shimmers. If you place a drop of water in the pan and it sizzles, you are ready to cook the fish.

Add the fish and cook on one side until browned (about five minutes). Gently flip and reduce the temperature to medium-low. Continue to cook, basting the fish with olive oil for another two to three minutes.

Plate fish, spoon relish over each piece, and garnish with fresh basil. Serve immediately. Serves four.

Black Bean Posole

    1 large onion, chopped

    3 poblano chilis, chopped

    6 cloves garlic, minced

    8 cups vegetable broth

    1 pound dry black beans

    ¼ cup olive oil

    2 tablespoons chili powder

    1 tablespoon tomato paste

    1 teaspoon dried oregano

    ¼ cup fresh lime juice (approximately two limes)

    1 teaspoon sea salt

    ⅛–¼ teaspoon cayenne pepper (depending on your taste buds)

    fresh cilantro, sliced avocado, and thinly sliced radishes

Sauté the onion, chilis, and garlic in olive oil until the onions are translucent. Pour into a large pot with a secure lid or a slow cooker. Add broth, chili powder, tomato paste, oregano, and black beans. Cook on high if using a slow cooker; if using a cooktop, bring ingredients to a boil and then simmer. Whether you use a slow cooker or pot, cook for four to five hours, making sure the beans are tender.

For quick black bean posole, you can substitute four sixteen-ounce cans or two twenty-eight-ounce cans of black beans for the one pound of dry beans. Cooking time will be less. After sautéing onions, add broth, chili powder, tomato paste, oregano, and beans to a large pot. Bring to a boil and simmer for thirty minutes stirring occasionally.

Stir in lime juice, salt, and cayenne. Top with cilantro, avocado, and radishes. Serves eight.

Miso-Glazed Sea Bass

⅓ cup mirin (Japanese rice wine)

⅔ cup sake

4 tablespoons soy sauce

⅓ cup miso paste

4 four- to five-ounce fresh sea bass fillets, 1½ to 2 inches thick

2 tablespoons green onion, chopped

Whisk together mirin, sake, soy sauce, and miso paste in a bowl. Place sea bass in large resealable plastic bag. Pour half the marinade over sea bass and chill in the refrigerator for two to five hours. Arrange sea bass on a baking sheet. Take other half of marinade and place in small pan (it will be heated later and drizzled over cooked sea bass before serving). Preheat oven's broiler and place rack approximately six inches from heat source. Leave the oven door slightly open and broil for seven to ten minutes until fish flakes easily. Keep a careful watch over the fish because you don't want to overcook it. Drizzle extra heated marinade over the sea bass and sprinkle with chopped green onions. Serve with mashed cauliflower and roasted asparagus. Serves four.

Meatless Bolognese

    1 medium onion, chopped

    1 thirteen-ounce package Gardein's ground "meat"

    15 ounces tomato sauce

    28 ounces diced tomatoes

    1 green bell pepper, chopped

    2 cloves garlic, minced

    8 ounces of either white or Baby Bella mushrooms, sliced

    4 tablespoons olive oil

    1 tablespoon oregano or 2 sprigs fresh basil, finely chopped

    1 teaspoon balsamic vinegar

    salt and pepper to taste

    vegan Parmesan (to sprinkle over pasta or peppers)*

In a pot, heat two tablespoons of olive oil over medium heat; sauté onions, peppers, mushrooms, and garlic until onions are translucent. Add tomato sauce, diced tomatoes, balsamic vinegar, and oregano or basil. Bring to a boil and then simmer for thirty minutes. Five minutes before serving, heat the remaining two tablespoons of olive oil in a frying pan and brown the Gardein (stirring often so it doesn't burn). Salt and pepper to taste. Combine marinara sauce with the browned Gardein and mix well before serving. Serves four.

*This Bolognese can be served over brown rice pasta or as a filler for stuffed green peppers (core the peppers, fill with Bolognese, and bake for thirty minutes [or until peppers are soft] in a 350° oven).

Desserts

Chia Seed Pudding

2 cups unsweetened almond, coconut, or cashew milk (I like almond)

7 tablespoons chia seeds

½ teaspoon vanilla extract

Stir intermittently for ten to fifteen minutes to avoid clumping. Cover with plastic wrap and refrigerate overnight. Spoon into serving dishes and finish off with black berries, sliced strawberries, or shaved dark chocolate. Serves four to six, depending on the size of the serving dishes.

Chocolate Red Devil Brownies

This recipe is adapted from Joanne Stepaniak's *The Vegan Sourcebook*.[2]

2 cups whole wheat pastry flour or barley flour

¼ cup coconut sugar (organic; coconut sugar is unrefined and low glycemic)

½ cup unsweetened cocoa powder

1 teaspoon cinnamon

2 teaspoons double-acting baking powder

2 teaspoons baking soda

2 tablespoons flaxseed meal

1⅓ cups water

1 large beet, cooked and diced (1 cup)

⅓ cup applesauce

2 teaspoons apple cider vinegar

2 teaspoons vanilla extract

Preheat oven to 350°.

In a large mixing bowl, place flour, sugar, cocoa powder, cinnamon, baking powder, and baking soda and whisk until combined.

Place flaxseed meal in a dry blender. Add ⅓ cup water and blend about thirty seconds, until mixture is gummy. Add beets, remaining water, applesauce, vinegar, and vanilla and process for one to two minutes, until frothy and well blended.

Mix liquid into dry ingredients. Stir until combined, and then quickly spoon batter into buttered 13 × 9 pan.

Bake thirty-five to forty minutes, until toothpick inserted in the center comes out clean. Cool. Cut into squares. You can freeze by wrapping individually.

Serve brownies with a scoop of vanilla coconut-milk ice cream or nondairy almond-milk whip (Reddi makes one).

Final Thoughts

C hange is difficult. The status quo is comfortable and safe. It is understandable that the unfamiliar is scary and distressing and heightens suspicion. Routines, habits, and preconceived thoughts feel more comfortable, even though they may be unhealthy and destructive. When we put that first foot forward, when we open our minds to change, we give ourselves permission to explore what is possible instead of what is.

I am in awe of individuals who were stuck in what they thought was their destiny only to discover in their quest for happiness and health that their bodies responded to their courageous transformation. Fresh options, looking at their situation from a different perspective, and the willingness to try the practice of self-health all helped them in the long run.

I hope you will find something in *Forget Dieting!* to stimulate independent thought. Think outside the box and consider a change in the way you currently eat and live. Even though you may have had negative experiences with dieting in the past, the beauty of *Forget Dieting!* is that it's a lifestyle of fueling, not dieting. By knowing the rules of DDF, you will have a better understanding that daily eating is really about providing your body—your organic machine—with the necessary nutrition to operate at an optimal level and sustain life. Your mouth is NOT supposed to have a party at every meal!

You only have one life to live, as the saying goes. Repeating the same mistakes over and over again and expecting a different outcome is the definition of insanity. If you know that a chocolate donut is unhealthy for your machine, why would you want to eat one? Get out of your own way and make yourself a priority. Cherish, love, and protect your organic machine. You can do this! Don't tiptoe—jump into your *Forget Dieting!* lifestyle with both feet. I'm here to help you. Give *Forget Dieting!* a try. You have nothing to lose except weight and poor health.

Notes

Preface

1. "The U.S. Weight Loss & Diet Control Market," Marketresearch .com, May 2017, https://www.marketresearch.com/Marketdata -Enterprises-Inc-v416/Weight-Loss-Diet-Control-10825677.

2. Traci Mann et al., "Medicare's Search for Effective Obesity Treatments: Diets Are Not the Answer," *American Psychologist* 62, no. 3 (2007): 220–33. doi:10.1037/0003-066x.62.3.220.

Note to the Reader

1. "New Findings on Obesity and Cancer," ASCO Connection, February 4, 2019, https://connection.asco.org/blogs/new-findings-obesity -and-cancer.

2. "Cancer Prevention and Early Detection Facts & Figures 2019–2020," American Cancer Society, https://www.cancer.org/content/dam/cancer-org/research/cancer-facts-and-statistics/cancer-prevention-and-early-detection-facts-and-figures/cancer-prevention-and-early-detection-facts-and-figures-2019-2020.pdf.

3. "Facts about Childhood Obesity," Partnership for a Healthier America, http://www.ahealthieramerica.org/articles/facts-about -childhood-obesity-102.

Chapter 1

1. Clayton Thomas, MD, ed., *Taber's Cyclopedic Medical Dictionary* (Philadelphia: F. A. Davis Company, 1970).

2. Osler W. William Beaumont, "A Pioneer American Physiologist," *JAMA* 39 (1902): 1223–31.

3. Shirley Hawke Gragg, RN, BSN, and Olive Rees, RN, MA, *Scientific Principles in Nursing* (Saint Louis, MO: C. V. Mosby Company, 1970).

Chapter 2

1. "Report of the Commission on Ending Childhood Obesity. Implementation Plan: Executive Summary," WHO/NMH/PND/ECHO/17.1 (Geneva: World Health Organization, 2016), https://apps .who.int/iris/bitstream/handle/10665/259349/WHO-NMH-PND -ECHO-17.1-eng.pdf.

2. "Genetic Testing for Hereditary Cancer Syndromes," National Cancer Institute, https://www.cancer.gov/about-cancer/causes -prevention/genetics/genetic-testing-fact-sheet.

Chapter 3

1. Harvard Health Publishing, "Obesity: Unhealthy and Unmanly," Harvard Health, https://www.health.harvard.edu/mens-health/ obesity-unhealthy-and-unmanly.

2. "More Than 1 in 20 US Children and Teens Have Anxiety or Depression," *ScienceDaily*, April 24, 2018, https://www.sciencedaily .com/releases/2018/04/180424184119.htm.

Chapter 5

1. "U.S. News' 41 Best Diets Overall," *U.S. News & World Report*, January 2, 2019, https://health.usnews.com/wellness/food/slideshows/ best-diets-overall.

2. A. Friedman, "High-Protein Diets: Potential Effects on the Kidney in Renal Health and Disease," National Center for Biotechnology Information, December 2004, https://www.ncbi.nlm.nih.gov/ pubmed/15558517.

Chapter 8

1. John Vidal, "10 Ways Vegetarianism Can Help Save the Planet," *Guardian*, July 2010.

2. "Meat and the Environment," PETA, https://www.peta.org/issues/animals-used-for-food/meat-environment/2019.

Chapter 9

1. J. Donahoe, "Edward L. Thorndike: The Selectionist Connectionist," *Journal of the Experimental Analysis of Behavior* 72, no. 3 (1999): 451–54. doi:10.1901/jeab.1999.72-451.

2. Jane E. Brody, "The Science of Dieting: A Fight against Mind and Metabolism," *New York Times*, February 24, 1981, https://www.nytimes.com/1981/02/24/science/the-science-of-dieting-a-fight-against-mind-and-metabolism-027182.html.

3. Samantha M. McEvedy et al., "Ineffectiveness of Commercial Weight-Loss Programs for Achieving Modest but Meaningful Weight Loss: Systematic Review and Meta-analysis," *Journal of Health Psychology* 22, no. 12 (2017): 1614–27. doi:10.1177/1359105317705983.

4. Julia Steinberger and Stephen R. Daniels, "Obesity, Insulin Resistance, Diabetes, and Cardiovascular Risk in Children," *Circulation* 107, no. 10 (2003): 1448–53. doi:10.1161/01.cir.0000060923.07573.f2.

5. Angela Kaye Wooton and Lynne M. Melchior, "Obesity and Type 2 Diabetes in Our Youth: A Recipe for Cardiovascular Disease," *Journal for Nurse Practitioners* 13, no. 3 (2017): 222–27. doi:10.1016/j.nurpra.2016.08.035.

6. Loretta Graziano Breuning, *Habits of a Happy Brain* (Avon, MA: Adams Media, 2016).

Chapter 11

1. Javaheri Sogol, MD, MPH, and Susan Redline, MD, MPH, "Insomnia and Risk of Cardiovascular Disease," *Chest* (August 2017): 435–44.

2. Camila Hirotsu, Dergio Tufik, and Monica Levy Andersen, "Interactions between Sleep, Stress, and Metabolism: From Physiological to Pathological Conditions," National Center for Biotechnology Information, September 28, 2015, https://www.ncbi.nlm.nih.gov/pmc/articles/PMC4688585.

3. Matthew Pase, PhD, "Less REM Sleep Tied to Greater Risk of Dementia," *Neurology*, August 23, 2017, https://www.aan.com/PressRoom/Home/PressRelease/1574#targetText=Less%20REM%20Sleep%20Tied%20to,the%20American%20Academy%20of%20Neurology.

4. Cari Romm, "Americans Are Getting Worse at Taking Sleeping Pills," *The Atlantic*, August 12, 2014, https://www.theatlantic.com/health/archive/2014/08/americans-are-getting-worse-at-taking-sleeping-pills/375935.

5. Jon Johnson, "How to Tell If Stress Is Affecting Your Sleep," *Medical News Today*, September 2018, https://www.medicalnewstoday.com/articles/322994.php.

6. "The Brain-Sleep Connection: GCBH Recommendations on Sleep and Brain Health," Global Council on Brain Health, a Collaborative from AARP, July 2016, https://doi.org/10.26419/pia.00014.001.

7. Sasha Brown, "Sleep Aid Gets a Nod from MIT Study," *MIT TechTalk* 49, no. 20 (March 9, 2005): 5.

8. Blake Bakkila, "Moon Milk Is the Trendy New Drink That Could Help You Fall Asleep Faster," *Health Magazine*, June 15, 2018.

Chapter 12

1. Elizabeth Gilbert, *Eat, Pray, Love: One Woman's Search for Everything* (Oxford: Oxford University Press, 2014).

Chapter 13

1. Sean Esteban McCabe et al., "Non-medical Use of Prescription Stimulants among US College Students: Prevalence and Correlates from a National Survey," Society for the Study of Addiction, Wiley Online Library, December 10, 2004, https://doi.org/10.1111/j.1360-0443.2005.00944.x.

2. American College of Obstetricians and Gynecologists, "Committee Opinion No. 722: Marijuana Use during Pregnancy and Lactation," *Obstetrics & Gynecology* 130, no. 4 (October 2017): e207.

3. R. W. Foltin, M. W. Fischman, and M. F. Byren, "Effects of Smoked Marijuana on Food Intake and Body Weight of Human Living in a Residential Laboratory," Department of Psychiatry and Behavioral Science, Johns Hopkins University School of Medicine, Baltimore, Maryland, August 1988.

4. S. Cains et al., "Agrp Neuron Activity Is Required for Alcohol-Induced Overeating," *Nature Communications* 8 (2017). doi: 10.1038/ncomms14014.

Chapter 14

1. Herbert M. Shelton, *Food Combining Made Easy* (San Antonio, TX: Willow Pub., 1984); William Howard Hay, *Hay Diet; Pocket Guide*, comp. Edward H. Dengel (New York: n.p., 1934).

Chapter 22

1. Deborah Madison, *Vegetarian Cooking for Everyone* (New York: Broadway Books, 2007), 381.

2. Joanne Stepaniak, *The Vegan Sourcebook* (Los Angeles, CA: Lowell House, 1998), 314.

Bibliography

"American College of Endocrinology Consensus Statement on Guidelines for Glycemic Control*." *Endocrine Practice* 8, Supplement 1 (2002): 5–11. doi:10.4158/ep.8.s1.5.

American College of Obstetricians and Gynecologists. "Committee Opinion No. 722: Marijuana Use during Pregnancy and Lactation." *Obstetrics & Gynecology* 130, no. 4 (October 2017): e205–e209.

Bakkila, Blake. "Moon Milk Is the Trendy New Drink That Could Help You Fall Asleep Faster." *Health Magazine*. June 15, 2018.

Beaumont, Osler W. William. "A Pioneer American Physiologist." *JAMA* 39 (1902): 1223–31.

"The Brain-Sleep Connection: GCBH Recommendations on Sleep and Brain Health." Global Council on Brain Health, a Collaborative from AARP. July 2016. https://doi.org/10.26419/pia.00014.001.

Brody, Jane E. "The Science of Dieting: A Fight against Mind and Metabolism." *New York Times*. February 24, 1981. https://www.nytimes.com/1981/02/24/science/the-science-of-dieting-a-fight-against-mind-and-metabolism-027182.html.

Brown, Sasha. "Sleep Aid Gets a Nod from MIT Study." *MIT TechTalk* 49, no. 20 (March 9, 2005): 5.

Cains, S., C. Blomeley, M. Kollo, R. Racz, and D. Burdakov. "Agrp Neuron Activity Is Required for Alcohol-Induced Overeating." *Nature Communications* 8 (2017). doi: 10.1038/ncomms14014.

"Cancer Prevention and Early Detection Facts & Figures 2019–2020." American Cancer Society. https://www.cancer.org/content/dam/cancer-org/research/cancer-facts-and-statistics/cancer-prevention-and-early-detection-facts-and-figures/cancer

-prevention-and-early-detection-facts-and-figures-2019-2020
.pdf.

Donahoe, J. "Edward L. Thorndike: The Selectionist Connectionist." *Journal of the Experimental Analysis of Behavior* 72, no. 3 (1999): 451–54. doi:10.1901/jeab.1999.72-451.

"Facts about Childhood Obesity." Partnership for a Healthier America. http://www.ahealthieramerica.org/articles/facts-about-childhood -obesity-102.

Foltin, R. W., M. W. Fischman, and M. F. Byren. "Effects of Smoked Marijuana on Food Intake and Body Weight of Human Living in a Residential Laboratory." Department of Psychiatry and Behavioral Science, Johns Hopkins University School of Medicine, Baltimore, Maryland, August 1988.

Friedman, A. "High-Protein Diets: Potential Effects on the Kidney in Renal Health and Disease." National Center for Biotechnology Information. December 2004. https://www.ncbi.nlm.nih.gov/ pubmed/15558517.

"Genetic Testing for Hereditary Cancer Syndromes." National Cancer Institute. https://www.cancer.gov/about-cancer/causes-prevention/ genetics/genetic-testing-fact-sheet.

Gilbert, Elizabeth. *Eat, Pray, Love: One Woman's Search for Everything.* Oxford: Oxford University Press, 2014.

Gragg, Shirley Hawke, RN, BSN, and Olive Rees, RN, MA. *Scientific Principles in Nursing.* Saint Louis, MO: C. V. Mosby Company, 1970.

Graziano Breuning, Loretta. *Habits of a Happy Brain.* Avon, MA: Adams Media, 2016.

Hay, William Howard. *Hay Diet; Pocket Guide.* Comp. Edward H. Dengel. New York: n.p., 1934.

Hirotsu, Camila, Dergio Tufik, and Monica Levy Andersen. "Interactions between Sleep, Stress, and Metabolism: From Physiological to Pathological Conditions." National Center for Biotechnology Information. September 28, 2015. https://www.ncbi.nlm.nih.gov/ pmc/articles/PMC4688585.

Johnson, Jon. "How to Tell If Stress Is Affecting Your Sleep." *Medical News Today.* September 2018. https://www.medicalnewstoday .com/articles/322994.php.

Madison, Deborah. *Vegetarian Cooking for Everyone*. New York: Broadway Books, 2007.

Mann, Traci, A. Janet Tomiyama, Erika Westling, Ann-Marie Lew, Barbara Samuels, and Jason Chatman. "Medicare's Search for Effective Obesity Treatments: Diets Are Not the Answer." *American Psychologist* 62, no. 3 (2007): 220–33. doi:10.1037/0003-066x.62.3.220.

McCabe, Sean Esteban, et al. "Non-medical Use of Prescription Stimulants among US College Students: Prevalence and Correlates from a National Survey." Society for the Study of Addiction. Wiley Online Library. December 10, 2004. https://doi.org/10.1111/j.1360-0443.2005.00944.x.

McEvedy, Samantha M., Gillian Sullivan-Mort, Siân A. McLean, Michaela C. Pascoe, and Susan J. Paxton. "Ineffectiveness of Commercial Weight-Loss Programs for Achieving Modest but Meaningful Weight Loss: Systematic Review and Meta-analysis." *Journal of Health Psychology* 22, no. 12 (2017): 1614–27. doi:10.1177/1359105317705983.

"Meat and the Environment." PETA. https://www.peta.org/issues/animals-used-for-food/meat-environment/2019.

"Mental Well-Being." AARP. https://doi.org/10.26419/pia.00037.001.

"More Than 1 in 20 US Children and Teens Have Anxiety or Depression." *ScienceDaily*. April 24, 2018. https://www.sciencedaily.com/releases/2018/04/180424184119.htm.

"New Findings on Obesity and Cancer." ASCO Connection. February 4, 2019. https://connection.asco.org/blogs/new-findings-obesity-and-cancer.

"Obesity: Unhealthy and Unmanly." Harvard Health. https://www.health.harvard.edu/mens-health/obesity-unhealthy-and-unmanly.

Pase, Matthew, PhD. "Less REM Sleep Tied to Greater Risk of Dementia." *Neurology*. August 23, 2017. https://www.aan.com/PressRoom/Home/PressRelease/1574#targetText=Less%20REM%20Sleep%20Tied%20to,the%20American%20Academy%20of%20Neurology.

"Report of the Commission on Ending Childhood Obesity. Implementation Plan: Executive Summary." WHO/NMH/PND/ECHO/17.1. Geneva: World Health Organization, 2016. https://apps.who.int/

iris/bitstream/handle/10665/259349/WHO-NMH-PND-ECHO
-17.1-eng.pdf.

Romm, Cari. "Americans Are Getting Worse at Taking Sleeping
Pills." *The Atlantic.* August 12, 2014. https://www.theatlantic.com/
health/archive/2014/08/americans-are-getting-worse-at-taking
-sleeping-pills/375935.

Rosen, Candice. *The Pancreatic Oath.* Chicago: Candice Rosen Health
Counseling, 2011.

Shelton, Herbert M. *Food Combining Made Easy.* San Antonio, TX:
Willow Pub., 1984.

Sogol, Javaheri, MD, MPH, and Susan Redline, MD, MPH. "Insomnia
and Risk of Cardiovascular Disease." *Chest* (August 2017): 435–44.

Steinberger, Julia, and Stephen R. Daniels. "Obesity, Insulin Resistance,
Diabetes, and Cardiovascular Risk in Children." *Circulation* 107,
no. 10 (2003): 1448–53. doi:10.1161/01.cir.0000060923.07573.f2.

Stepaniak, Joanne. *The Vegan Sourcebook.* Los Angeles, CA: Lowell
House, 1998.

Thomas, Clayton, MD, ed. *Taber's Cyclopedic Medical Dictionary.* Philadelphia: F. A. Davis Company, 1970.

"U.S. News' 41 Best Diets Overall." *U.S. News & World Report.* January 2, 2019. https://health.usnews.com/wellness/food/slideshows/
best-diets-overall.

"The U.S. Weight Loss & Diet Control Market." Marketresearch
.com. May 2017. https://www.marketresearch.com/Marketdata
-Enterprises-Inc-v416/Weight-Loss-Diet-Control-10825677.

Vidal, John. "10 Ways Vegetarianism Can Help Save the Planet."
Guardian. July 2010.

Wooton, Angela Kaye, and Lynne M. Melchior. "Obesity and Type 2
Diabetes in Our Youth: A Recipe for Cardiovascular Disease." *Journal for Nurse Practitioners* 13, no. 3 (2017): 222–27. doi:10.1016/j
.nurpra.2016.08.035.

Index

absorption, 3, 5, 6

accountability, 125

ACE. *See* angiotensin-converting enzyme inhibitors

acid solutions, 104

addiction: drugs and alcohol, 96–100; to food, 66; healthy, 75

adipose cells (fat cells), 10, 15, 17, 18, 22, 24, 135

adipose tissue, 74

adjustment phenomenon, 41

adrenal glands, 16, 22, 76

adrenaline, 16, 18, 22, 25

Adrenobesity™, 18–20

alcohol, 10, 24, 85, 86; absorption of, 5; addiction, 96–100; blood glucose and, 99; in college, 97; drugs and, 96–100; obesity and, 98; water and, 99, 146, 147; wine, 47, 52, 95, 98, 99, 117, 121, 147

alkaline solutions, 104

alpha-blockers, 80

American Cancer Society, xvii

American Society of Clinical Oncology, xvii

amylase, 4

androgens, 18

angiotensin-converting enzyme (ACE) inhibitors, 81

angiotensin II-receptor blockers (ARBs), 81

animal(s), 118; agriculture, 54; on factory farms, 54; protein, 35–36, 46, 54–55, 60, 70, 93, 103, 105, *106*, 112, 114, 134; suffering of, 54

antibiotics, 55

antihistamines, 81

anxiety, xvii, 20

appetite, 15, 17, 20, 22, 45, 83, 98

appetizers, recipes for, 151–52

apple cider vinegar cleanse drink, 53, 54, 149

ARBs. *See* angiotensin II-receptor blockers

arteries, plaque build-up in, 9

asthma, 63

atherosclerosis, 8, 9

Atkins diet, 35
attitude, 60, 61, 82, 93

basics, of eating: glucose and
    insulin effects, 8–14, *9, 11*;
    hormones, stress, and weight,
    15–25, 74; process of, 3–7
Beaumont, William, 4
behavior modification, 24; in
    DDF, 59–71; goals for, 67–71;
    most effective techniques for,
    71; objectiveness in, 67; tools,
    93; transformation and, 25;
    weight loss and, 59
behavior therapy, 59
benign prostatic hyperplasia, 80
beta-blockers, 81
bicarbonate, 6
biking, 76
bio-individuality, xv, 36, 45, 114,
    125
biotin, 140
blood glucose, xi, 6, 36; adjust-
    ment phenomenon, 41;
    alcohol and, 99; continuous
    monitoring, 38–39; drugs
    and, 99; effects of, 8–14,
    9, 11; excess, 8; fasting, xv,
    44; glucometer, xiv, 34, *37,*
    37–38, 133; glucose tolerance,
    63; hyperglycemia, xiii, *9,*
    133–35; hypoglycemia, 33,
    39–40, 42, 53, 117, 122; levels,
    xiv, 53; meal discovery cards
    and, 127–32; monitoring of,
    37–41; NCDs and, 8; restau-
    rant meals and, 134; stress

and, 133; testing during DDF,
    30–31, 37–41, 45; weight gain
    and, xiii
blood pressure: high, xiii, xvii,
    8, 10, 12, 33, 63; medication,
    33, 60
bloodstream: adrenaline and
    cortisol in, 16; food particles
    in, 105; glucose and, 6–7, 12,
    45; glycogen and, 15; nutrient
    absorption into, 6; T cells in,
    138
blue light, 79
body: chemistry, xiv; composi-
    tion, xiv; dysmorphia, xvii;
    listening to, 31; positivity,
    xviii; respect for, 32
body-fat distribution, 15
bowel movement, 6, 135
bowling, 76
boxing, 76
brain, 78, 79
breakfast, 50; choices, 119–20;
    at college, 145; recipes for,
    152–55; during travel, 146
Breuning, Loretta Graziano, 67

caffeine, 24, 82, 85
calcium, 16, 46, 137, 140
calendar, DDF, 52–55, *55,* 70,
    147
calories, 135; burning of, 76;
    counting of, xii, 46, 133;
    excess of, 10; zero, 45
cancer, 14, 46, 59, 99; breast,
    xiii–xv; causes of, xvii; City of
    Hope Comprehensive Cancer

Center, xiii–xv; incidence of, 12; obesity and, xvii, 14
carbohydrates, 5, 10, 40, 103, 109, 134; counting of, xii, 46; intake of, 35. *See also* diets
cardiovascular disease, 60
carotenoids, 139
Cayce, Edgar, 103
cell phone apps, for diet, exercise, and diabetes, 125–26
Centers for Disease Control, xvii
chemical imbalances, 105
childhood obesity, xviii, 13, 63
cholesterol, xv; guidelines, *11*; heart and, 36; high, xiii, 8–10, 12, 63, 67
cholinesterase inhibitors, 81
circadian rhythm, 79
City of Hope Comprehensive Cancer Center, xiii–xv
classical conditioning, 59
climate change, 54
coenzyme Q10, 137
cognitive abilities, 80
cognitive restructuring, 71
college: DDF at, 144–46; meals at, 144–46; overdoses and alcohol at, 97; stress at, 145; weight gain at, 145
combinations, of food. *See* food combining
congestive heart failure, 65, 81
contingency planning, 71
continuous glucose monitoring, 38–39. *See also* blood glucose
coping mechanisms, 96
coronary heart disease, xvii

corticosteroids, 81
cortisol, 15, 21, 25, 74; fight-or-flight response, 16, 22; weight loss and, 16
cruise ships, 147

dairy, 46, 112
dancing, 76
Data-Driven Fueling (DDF), xi, xiii, 14, 17, 27–28; basic principles of, 29–31; behavior modification in, 59–71; blood glucose monitoring for, 37–41; calendar, 52–55, *55*, 70, 147; during college, 144–46; daily schedule for, 49–51; eating less in, 30; food combining, basic, 103–10, *106*; foods to avoid with, 31–32; guidelines, 29–32; healthy addictions and, 75; insulin and, 42–43, 49, 60, 89; lifestyle, 33–43; listening to your body with, 31; meal anatomy of, 111–18; meal choices, 119–24; meal schedule for, 48–49; measurements prior to, 34; movement and, 30, 72–77; program, 44–47; sabotage and, 88–95; sleep and, 78–87; splurging in, 52–53; testing for, 30–31, 37–41; during travel, 146–48; tuning in to, 30–31, 41–43; unhealthy temptations and, 31; weekly schedule for, 115–17

Davis, Donald, 137
DDF. *See* Data-Driven Fueling
deep breathing, 23, 51
dehydration, 134
dementia, 80
depression, xvii, 20, 60
desserts, recipes for, 165–66. *See
    also* sweets
diabetes, 35, 81, 84, 89, 125. *See
    also* type 1 diabetes; type 2
    diabetes
diets, 21; Atkins, 35; cell phone
    apps for, 125–26; Dukan, 35;
    failures of, reasons for, 143;
    Keto, 35; lifestyle and, 34;
    low-carb, 35; Paleo, 35; serial,
    60; short-term, 36; South
    Beach, 35; types of, 35; yo-yo,
    60
digestion, 3–4, 105, 109, 143
digestive energy, 104
digestive enzymes, 5
digestive tract, 3–4
dinner, 51; choices, 123–24;
    at college, 146; recipes for,
    159–64
dreams, 79. *See also* sleep
drowsiness, 78–79, 81
drugs, 96–100
Dukan diet, 35

eating: ethnic, 64–65; out of
    element, 144–48; process of,
    3–7; stress/emotional, 112.
    See also basics, of eating
The Enemy Within (Firestone),
    92

Environmental Protection
    Agency, 54
enzymes, 5–6, 103–5
epiglottis, 4
esophagus, 3–4
estrogen, 18
ethnic eating, 64–65
exercise. *See* movement

fainting, 122
family obesity, 65
famine, 142
fast food, 64
fat cells. *See* adipose cells
fats: counting of, xii, 46; healthy,
    110, 114; storage of, 18,
    134
fatty liver disease, 63
fermentation, in stomach, 46,
    105, 109
fight-or-flight response, 16, 22.
    See also cortisol
Firestone, Robert, 92
fish oil, 137
fluid retention, 146, 148
folic acid, 139
food: addiction to, 66; behaviors
    around, 61; eating less, 30; as
    fuel, 29, 65, 118, 167; healthy
    choices of, xiv, 7; processed,
    112; as reward, 91; self-sooth-
    ing with, 22; unwise choices
    of, 8; vitamins from, 137;
    white, 45, 112
food combining, 47; basic,
    103–10, *106*; proper, *113*;
    during travel, 148

Food Combining Made Easy
(Shelton), 103
food sensitivities, 105
fruits, 46, *106*, 107; dried, 47,
114; eaten alone, 112
fuel: food as, 29, 65, 118, 167;
using excess, 135. *See also*
Data-Driven Fueling

gallbladder disease, xvii
garlic, 138
gastric juices, 4
gastroesophageal reflux disease, 80
gastrointestinal tract, 143. *See
also* digestion
Gilbert, Elizabeth, 93
glucagon, 5–6, 7
glucometer, xiv, 34, *37*, 37–38,
133. *See also* continuous
glucose monitoring; Data-
Driven Fueling
glucosamine/chondroitin, 81
glucose. *See* blood glucose
glucose tolerance, 63
Glucotrol, 45
glycogen, 6, 15, 134
goals: for behavior modification,
67–71; breaking down, 141;
long-term, 61; self-sabotage
and, 93; smaller, 141; weekly,
70
gratitude, 118
green juice recipe, 150

habits, healthy, 48, 75
Habits of a Happy Brain (Breuning), 67

Hay, William Howard, 103
The Hay Diet (Hay), 103
HDL. *See* high-density
lipoprotein
health: drugs and alcohol,
96–100; behavior modifi-
cation, 59–71; movement,
72–77; sabotage, 88–95; sleep,
78–87
heart disease, xii, xvii, 8–10, 36,
65, 81
hemoglobin A1c, xv, 13, 36
high-density lipoprotein (HDL),
10, *11*
hiking, 76
hormones, 55, 138; pancreatic, 5;
sex, 15, 17–20; stress, 15–16,
21–22, 74; weight and, 15–25
housework, 76
hula hooping, 75
Hung Chao-Ming, 80
hunger, 17, 42, 49, 83, 98
hyperglycemia, xiii, 9, 133–35
hyperinsulinemia, 16, 17–18, 42
hypoglycemia, 33, 39–40, 42, 53,
117, 122

immune system, 16, 81, 83, 138,
139
inactivity, 13, 60, 77. *See also*
movement
inflammation, 9, 22; chronic,
8–10; of joints, 138; of pancreas, 99
insomnia, 80, 82, 84, 85, 87
insulin, 35; bodily response to, 7;
DDF and, 42–43, 49, 60, 89;

effects of, 8–14, *9, 11*; fluctuations in, xiv; glucometer, xiv, 34, *37*, 37–38, 133; high levels of, 8, *9*; hyperinsulinemia, 16, 17–18, 42; leptin and, 15, 17; NCDs and, 8; overproduction of, 22; production of, 5, 6–7; resistance, xiii, xiv, 7, 12, 13, 84; sex hormones and, 15, 17–20, *19. See also* blood glucose; type 1 diabetes

interstitial fluid, 38

iron, 137

journal, 51, 70, 125–27

Journal of the American College of Nutrition, 137

juice, 47, 53; cleanse, 54; green, 150; Montmorency Tart Cherry, 138

jumping jacks, 76

jump rope, 76

Keto diet, 35

ketones, 35

ketosis, 35

kidneys, 12, 35, 76

large intestine, 3

LDL. *See* low-density lipoprotein

leptin, 15, 17. *See also* hormones

lifestyle: change, 48, 60, 126, 135; diets and, 34; quality of, xiv. *See also* Data-Driven Fueling

light sleep, 79

liquid fast, 53, 135; recipes for, 149–51

liver, 5

Li Ying-Chun, 80

low-density lipoprotein (LDL), 10, *11*

lunch, 51; choices, 121–22; at college, 145; recipes for, 155–58; during travel, 147

lymphocytes, 138

macronutrients, 103

magnesium, 137, 140

marijuana, 97, 145

marketing, 63

McEvedy, Samantha, 62

meal: anatomy of, 111–18; choices, 119–24; gratitude for, 118; as medicine, 111; planning of, 119–24, 127–32; schedule, 48–49, 114, 115–17; time approximations for, 114

meal discovery cards, 51, 127–32

measurements, prior to DDF, 34

medications: ACE inhibitors, 81; alpha-blockers, 80; antibiotics, 55; ARBs, 81; beta-blockers, 81; cholinesterase inhibitors, 81; coenzyme Q10, 137; corticosteroids, 81; glucosamine/chondroitin, 81; Glucotrol, 45; for high blood pressure, 33, 60; hypoglycemia and, 117; lowering dosages of, 60; melatonin, 79, 85–86; Metformin, xii, 45; multivitamin, 137; nonsedating H1 antagonists (antihistamines), 81; prescription,

53, 67; side effects of, 117; for sleep, 80, 82, 84, 85–86; SSRIs, 81; statin drugs, 10, *11*, 81; weight gain and, 84. *See also* vitamin(s)

meditation, 24, 50, 85

melatonin, 79, 85–86

memory consolidation, 78

menu planning, 119–24, 127–32

metabolic syndrome, xiii, 12, 18, 63

metabolism, 15

Metformin, xii, 45

methane, 54

Montmorency Tart Cherry Juice, 138

moon milk, 86–87

mouth, 3–4

movement, xiv, 21, 30, 51, 72–77; daily, 73; enjoyment of, 73; for excess fuel, 135; after meals, 135; stress and, 74

multivitamin, 137. *See also* vitamin(s)

muscle: abdominal, 75; build-up of, 74; corticosteroids and, 81; memory, 23; movement and, 30, 74; sleep and, 79; use of, 77

naps, 83

natural sugars, 105

negativity, 68, 93

noncommunicable diseases (NCDs), xiii, 12–13; causes of, 43; glucose and insulin with, 8; medication for, 80;

reversal of, 61, 71; weight gain and, 43

non-rapid eye movement (NREM) sleep, 79

nonsedating H1 antagonists (antihistamines), 81

nutrition, 103, 167; for children, 13; content, 137; counseling for, xv; culturally sensitive, xv; label, 54; PNP, xiii–xv; poor, 16; precision, xi, 34, 70

nuts, 108, 109, 114, 147

obesity, 8; *Adrenobesity*™, 18–20; alcohol and, 98; behavior and, 59; cancer and, xvii, 14; in childhood, xviii, 13, 63; epidemic, xviii; family, 65; leptin and, 15, 17; mobility and, 60; prevention of, 14; rates of, xvii, 20; self-esteem and, 68; sleep and, 80; stress and, 15–16

objectiveness, in behavior modification, 67

omega-3 fatty acids, 137

opioid crisis, 97. *See also* drugs

organic machine, body as, 34, 91

osteoarthritis, xvii, 60

pain, xvii, 66, 96; back, 60; joint, 60, 81; response to, 15

Paleo diet, 35

pancreas, 6, 111; abuse of, xiii; adjustment phenomenon and, 41; foods for, xv; function of, xii; hormones,

5; hyperinsulinemia and, 16, 17–18, 42; inflammation of, 99; insulin resistance and, xiii, xiv, 7, 12, 13, 84; leptin and, 15, 17; protection of, xiii, 21, 23, 30, 36, 73, 77, 89, 135; vitamins and, 136; weight gain and, xiii
pancreatic duct, 6
Pancreatic Nutrition Program (PNP), xiii–xv
The Pancreatic Oath, xi
pantothenic acid, 140
Pase, Matthew, 80
Pavlov, Ian, 59
pepsin, 103
pharynx, 4
phosphorus, 137
physical activity. *See* movement
Pilates, 76
plaque, 9
plateaus, in weight loss, 141–43
PNP. *See* Pancreatic Nutrition Program
points, counting of, xii
pollution, 54–55
polycystic ovarian syndrome, xiii, 12
positive reinforcement, 71
potassium, 140
problem solving, 71
programmed learning, 59
protein, 137, 142; animal, 35, 36, 46, 54, 55, 60, 70, 93, 103, 105, *106*, 112, 114, 134; plant-based, 46, 105, *106*; powder, 112; starch and, 112

ptyalin, 103
public health, 55, 97
pulmonary embolism, 10
punishment, 59, 72

rapid eye movement (REM) sleep, 79
Raynaud's disease, 80
recipes: appetizers/snacks, 151–52; breakfast, 152–55; desserts, 165–66; dinner, 159–64; liquid fasts, 149–51; lunch, 155–58; multigenerational, 65
rectum, 3
reinforcement, 59, 66, 71
REM. *See* rapid eye movement sleep
renal disease, xiii, 12
restaurant: eating at, 64, 133–34; health-conscious, 121; meal choices at, 134; salt use at, 134, 146
riboflavin, 137

sabotage, 62, 88–95; self, 74, 92, 134; tips to reduce, 94
salivary glands, 4
scale, 44, 49, *50*, 134, 145
seeds, 109, 114
selective serotonin reuptake inhibitors (SSRIs), 81
selenium, 140
self-awareness, 125
self-blame, 68
self-care, 61, 77
self-esteem, 68

self-health, xiii, 61, 66, 167
self-love, xviii, 93
self-monitoring, 71. *See also*
    glucometer
self-sabotage, 74, 92, 134
sex hormones: insulin and, 15,
    17–20, *19*; weight gain and,
    18. *See also* hormones
Shelton, Herbert M., 103
Skinner, B. F., 59
sleep, 23, 51; apnea, xvii, 63, 80;
    deprivation, 80, 83; dreams
    and, 79; drowsiness, 78–79,
    81; importance of, 78–87;
    insomnia, 80, 82, 84, 85, 87;
    light, 79; medications for,
    80, 82, 84, 85–86; naps
    and, 83; NREM, 79; REM,
    79; restless, 80; stages of,
    78–79; stress and, 80, 82–83;
    tips for, 83–85; weight loss
    and, 87
small intestine, 3, 5, 6
smoothies, 46, 53–54, 109, 112,
    145; recipes, 150–51
Smooth Move Tea, 142
snacks, 51, 53, 54; calo-
    rie-friendly, 135; choices, 122;
    healthy, 43; meal discovery
    cards and, 127; recipes,
    151–52; schedule, 49, 114,
    115–17, 147
socioeconomics, 64
soda, 112
sodium, 140
South Beach diet, 35
squats, for movement, 75–76

SSRIs. *See* selective serotonin
    reuptake inhibitors
St. Martin, Alexis, 4
stamina, 77
starch, *106*, 107, 113–14
starvation mode, 98, 141
statin drugs, 10, *11*, 81
steps, counting of, xii, 74
Stevia, 45
stimulus control, 71
stomach, 3–4
stress: blood glucose and, 133;
    at college, 145; hormones,
    15–16, 21–22, 74; manage-
    ment, 21, 125, 126; reduction,
    16, 23–25; sleep and, 80,
    82–83; weight and, 8, 15–25;
    weight loss and, 22
stroke, xvii, 10, 80
sugar, 10, 53, 54, 112, 114, 147;
    low, 121; natural, 105; refined,
    45; withdrawal, 66. *See also*
    blood glucose
Super B complex, 137
Super Dieter's Tea, 142
sweeteners, artificial, 45–46
sweets, 112, 133, 165–66
swimming, 30, 76, 147

tape measure, 44
tart cherry concentrate, 138
T cells, 138
tea, 142–43, 147
temptations, 31, 61, 89, 93, 94
tennis, 76
testosterone, xiii, 12, 18, 19
Thorndike, Edward, 59

thymosin, 138
thymus, 138–39
transformation: behavior modification and, 25; health, 18, 48, 66, 90, 126, 167; inner, 71
travel, 146–48
triggers: identification of, 62, 70; for temptation, 31
triglycerides, xv, 7, 10, *11*, 12
trophology, 103
type 1 diabetes, 13
type 2 diabetes, xvii, 63; in children, 13–14; insulin resistance and, xiii, xiv, 7, 13, 84; sleep and, 80. *See also* blood glucose; pancreas
typhus, 97

vacation. *See* travel
valerian, 85, 86
vegetable(s), *106*, 142; list of, 108; non-starchy, 105, 110; oils, 140; as protein, 46; starchy, 40; vitamins and, 35, 137
vitamin(s), 51; A, 139; B1, 139; B2, 137, 139; B3, 139; B6, 139; B12, 140; basic supplementation of, 136; biotin, 140; C, 137, 140; calcium, 140; carotenoids, 139; coenzyme Q10, 137; D, 137, 140; with DDF and movement, 136; deficiencies, 35, 136; dosages of, 136; E, 140; fish oil, 137; folic acid, 139; food sources of, 139–40;

glucosamine/chondroitin, 81; K, 140; magnesium, 137, 140; pantothenic acid, 140; potassium, 140; prescription medications and, 136; selenium, 140; Super B complex, 137; supplements, 137–39; in vegetables, 35, 137; weight loss and, 136; zinc, 137, 140

waist circumference, xv, 19, 44, 146
walking: after meals, 135; for movement, 23–24, 30, 51, 73–74, 75, 77, 85, 142
water: alcohol and, 99, 146, 147; as beverage, 47, 53, 147; retention, 134; weight gain from, 146
weight gain, 7; at college, 145; fluid retention and, 146, 148; glucose and, xiii; hormones and, 15–25; leptin and, 15, 17; after loss, xii, 36, 62; medications and, 84; mobility and, 60; NCDs and, 43; pancreatic abuse and, xiii; polycystic ovarian syndrome and, xiii, 12; poor health and, 8, 71; risk for, 84; stress and, 8, 15–25; sweeteners and, 45; during travel, 146
weight lifting, 76
weight loss: affecting others, 90–91; behavior modification and, 59; control over, xix;

cortisol and, 16; frustration with, 60; goals, 63, 70–71; long-term, xi; market, xii; movement and, 72–77; NCD reversal with, 71; permanent, 61; quick, 62; sleep and, 87; stress and, 22; sudden, 22; sustainable, xi, xiv, 29, 34, 36; during travel, 147; vitamins and, 136. *See also* sabotage

wine, 47, 52, 95, 98, 99; with DDF, 117, 121, 147. *See also* alcohol
withdrawal symptoms, 66
workouts. *See* movement
World Health Organization, 99

yardwork, 76
yoga, 30, 51, 60, 76, 147

zinc, 137, 140

About the Author

Candice P. Rosen is a registered nurse and certified health coach with a master's degree in social work. Her experiences as a therapist and as a nurse give her a unique perspective when it comes to nutritional counseling. Candice believes in the practice of self-health. She is the author of *The Pancreatic Oath*, a book for health-conscious people searching for improved wellness and weight loss through diet and blood glucose regulation. She is also the creator of the Pancreatic Nutritional Program and Data-Driven Fueling. Both programs focus on precision nutrition.

In addition to completing her third book, *Forget Dieting!*, Rosen lectures on pancreatic abuse and the prevention and reversal of obesity and noncommunicable diseases. She maintains a private practice, Candice Rosen Health Counseling, in Los Angeles, California. She is married, the mother of four grown children, and the grandmother of one. She enjoys hiking, tennis, golf, horseback riding, swimming, entertaining, travel, and spending time with family and friends.